D0735744

Stutter
No
More

DR. MARTIN F. SCHWARTZ

Research Professor, New York University Medical Center

SIMON & SCHUSTER
New York   London   Toronto   Sydney   Tokyo   Singapore

Simon & Schuster
Simon & Schuster Building
Rockefeller Center
1230 Avenue of the Americas
New York, New York 10020

Designed by Irving Perkins Associates
Manufactured in the United States of America

10 9 8 7 6 5 4 3 2 1

Library of Congress Cataloging-in-Publication Data

ISBN 0-671-72612-9

Contents

6   *Contents*

15. For Parents: Will Your Child Outgrow
    the Problem?   88
16. Selecting a Treatment Program   95
17. Ongoing Research for Treatment   97

Part Three   SUCCESS STORIES

18. The Computer Professional   105
19. The Importer   110
20. The Seminary Student   112
21. The Retired Mechanical Engineer   116
22. The Social Worker   118

Part Four   FINAL WORDS

23. To the Stutterer   125
24. To Friends and Family   127
25. To the Therapist   130

Appendix

A Study of the Long-term Effects of a
    Multidimensional Treatment Program
    for Stutterers   135
Acknowledgments   139
Index   140

A Note to the Reader

As a clinician, I have always found dealing with speech problems to be a scientific and intellectual challenge. But even more, it has been a human concern. Whether undertaking basic research on birth defects such as cleft lip and palate, or investigating the more widespread and pervasive affliction of stuttering, I have discovered that these problems draw on the power of empathy as much as acumen.

Consider the following account of going through life as a stutterer. Many of you will see yourselves in this case history, or you'll recognize the frustrations expressed by people you know who stutter. Either way, you will understand why I feel so deeply about the problem and why I continue to work personally with stutterers whenever I can.

Imagine that from the time you were a child you stuttered with everyone. Not that you wanted to stutter, mind you; you just couldn't help yourself. As a result you often went to great lengths to avoid stuttering and, in so doing, found that people misunderstood you. They considered you aloof, withdrawn, a loner, the silent type.

But you ached to be with people, you had much to say, and the thought of the interaction was marvelous. And so each night before you went to sleep you prayed that this dreadful affliction would be gone. But it was not to be.

As a child you were sent to specialists who tried to show

you how to stop stuttering or how to stutter in less offensive ways. Sometimes you stopped with them, but as soon as you left their office your stuttering returned, and their suggestions, which earlier had worked so well, now failed miserably.

The stuttering demeaned you, it humiliated you, it destroyed your self-esteem. And often, when it was at its worst, as if to add insult to injury, people laughed at you, called you stupid, and never took you seriously at all.

In school if you had a question you wouldn't ask it. If you had to respond and couldn't speak the correct answer you'd give an incorrect one. In the cafeteria, you'd order what you could say rather than what you wanted. Anything to avoid the humiliation.

You studied hard, and since you were intelligent, you received excellent grades—as long as the grades were based on written exams. You lived in constant dread of required oral reports and begged your parents to ask your teachers to excuse you from them. Some teachers were sensitive, and made class participation easier. Others insisted that the way to overcome the problem was to force you to participate—and the memory of this nightmare persisted for years and made your struggling worse, not only in class, but everywhere.

You wanted to go to college, but dreaded the prospect of an interview. As a matter of fact, any sort of interview was a nightmare. Because of this, jobs were difficult and you were lucky to find an employer who would overlook your problem.

Dating was another torture: the very prospect filled you with terror. The first hint of a stutter seemed to destroy the evening instantly. Occasionally you met someone kind, a person who did not appear to be bothered by your problem, someone who looked beyond it to the person beneath. These were wonderful times.

And as you grew older you grew smarter; you learned tricks to avoid stuttering and chose an occupation you could perform without penalty, like accounting or engineering or computer programming or truck driving—activities that could be performed alone.

Your parents gave up. They no longer mentioned your affliction. It was as if it didn't exist. And your friends and acquaintances did the same. A massive conspiracy of denial gradually descended to protect you and them from a behavior too painful for anyone to acknowledge.

You tried alcohol and illegal drugs because you heard these sometimes worked. But not for you; they only made things worse, and you stopped. You tried tranquilizers, anticonvulsants, beta-blockers—anything modern medicine might suggest had the slightest possibility of helping. But again, nothing.

You joined a self-help group of people with your problem, but it was like looking into a mirror. You especially couldn't stand confronting those more severely afflicted than yourself; it suggested what might happen if your stuttering worsened.

To say that the stuttering affected your life would be the profoundest of understatements. It permeated your life and controlled it so insidiously that you often wondered whether a life like this should continue.

And so you gave up. You quit looking for an answer. You joined the conspiracy of denial and made the best of it.

Fortunately, this tale of woe is soon to be history. We are at a turning point in our work with stutterers. Not only do we have a technique that works, but one that works quickly, often in a matter of minutes, and stops stuttering completely. We have perfected the procedures for making this technique habitual, and have made remarkable strides in eliminating the fears associated with stuttering.

The future is promising. New research is shedding light on the inner workings of the brain: the neural center responsible for stuttering has been located. It seems more likely than ever that the twenty-first century will witness a cure.

But until then, we can stop stuttering with a simply learned technique which, after a short period of practice, can become a permanent, new habit.

It is clear that no one need stutter anymore!

Part I

UNDERSTANDING

1 *The Discovery of the Physical Cause*

My DISCOVERY of the physical cause of stuttering was a complete accident—one of those things that I never expected to happen but that nonetheless changed the direction of my professional life. In 1974, I was a professor of speech science at New York University Medical Center, helping design an operation to improve the speech of patients born with cleft palate. I was using an ultrasound device called a Sonagraph to study throat-movement patterns in cleft-palate patients slated for surgery. These patterns had to be analyzed in order for us to locate the place in the throat where a piece of tissue would be removed to close the hole in the roof of the mouth.

One of the patients stuttered, and the Sonagraph showed that his throat constricted forcefully before every stutter. The pattern was very regular, and I couldn't help wondering about the meaning of this curious event.

I called a speech pathologist to ask if he knew of any relationship between the throat constrictions and stuttering I had observed. He knew of none, he said, since speech pathologists had never before been able to look at the throat during speech. My ultrasonic scan represented something new.

Excited by the prospect of a new discovery, we arranged to see several stutterers for ultrasonic examination. Within two weeks I had examined five—and all displayed the same pattern of constrictions.

My initial observation confirmed thus far, I applied the Sonagraph to different places vertically on the neck to see if the throat constrictions varied in intensity. I discovered that the further down the throat, the more vigorous the constriction. When the Sonagraph was applied to the side of the stutterer's larynx (voice box) at the base of the neck, something unexpected happened: just before every stutter, the vocal cords rose slightly and then suddenly slammed together in a constriction even more violent than any seen in the throat. Here, it seemed, was the center of activity—the vocal cords, pressed together forcefully. Here was the physical event that seemed to determine whether a person spoke with a stutter or not.

In normal speech, the vocal cords are brought together by several pairs of muscles so that they touch each other very gently. The person then builds up air pressure beneath them by exhaling. When the air pressure becomes great enough, it blows the vocal cords apart, which sets them vibrating and makes sound. The sound is the raw material for speech production; it is converted into speech by movement of the lips, tongue, jaw, teeth, palate, and other articulators.

But in stutterers, for some reason, the vocal cords were pressed together so forcefully that the air required for speaking couldn't pass.

I proposed an explanation which seemed outlandish at the time, but has since been substantiated repeatedly by investigators; namely, that the physical source of all stuttering is a locking of the vocal cords. But at that time I still did not understand how a locking of the vocal cords could lead to the wide variety of speech struggles I observed in stutterers.

2 *The Hunt for the Stutter Reflex*

How COULD locked vocal cords produce such varied speech struggles? Speech therapists I spoke with maintained that there were three categories of stuttering: *hesitations* (sometimes called blockages), *repetitions* (of words, sounds, or syllables) and *prolongations* (again, of sounds or syllables). But this categorization seemed arbitrary and neglected many of the apparent differences I observed. Also, it related only to speech, completely disregarding the non-speech events that many stutterers exhibited.

Most speech pathologists nebulously conceptualized stuttering as an "incoordination" among respiratory, vocal-cord, and articulatory mechanisms. However, the precise nature of this incoordination was never spelled out and there seemed to be no research to support it. Why, if there was an "incoordination," did it disappear when the stutterer talked out loud to himself? And why was it not present continuously, but only on certain words?

After reviewing the literature, I remained convinced that the physical cause of stuttering lay at the vocal cords and that all the other behaviors observed were a reaction to the constriction of the vocal cords. But the precise nature of this response eluded me until one day, quite by accident, I found an answer.

There is a door in my office which I pass through each day. The routine is always the same. I go to the door, put my hand on the doorknob, turn it, pull the door open, walk through, and the door closes automatically behind me. It always works, I always expect it to work, and I'm never disappointed.

But one particular day a water pipe broke in the office above, and the water seeped slowly through the ceiling and into the wooden door. The door was swollen and stuck in the door frame, but I didn't know it because the seepage had been slow and I couldn't see it. So when I went to open the door, it didn't move; it was stuck. I pulled harder and harder until finally I wrenched the door open.

Twenty minutes later, I returned to the door and again found it stuck. I immediately yanked forcefully and it opened. At that instant I realized I had undergone a conditioning. I had learned, after just a single trial, to yank the door forcefully when I wanted to get it open. The fact that this initial struggle had resulted in success, meant that I had been rewarded for my efforts and thus, in the same situation, would likely struggle again. Which I did. I struggled with the door each time until it dried out and I could once again open it easily.

The incident gave me new insight into the stutter response, for the swollen door was quite like the locked vocal cords in a stutterer. Just as I had learned to struggle to open the door, it seemed logical that a stutterer would struggle to find ways to speak, and that he would then learn these ways—make them habitual—since they helped him achieve the desired result.

I thought back to some of the nonverbal behaviors stutterers used to facilitate fluency to see if they could be explained in light of this new understanding. For instance, some patients would suck air in quickly through their mouths just before speaking. Now this seemed to make sense. The more rapidly one inhales, the wider the vocal cords open to allow a greater volume of air to pass. The patients were using this rapid breathing-in to open their locked vocal cords so they could begin to speak before the cords locked again.

Similarly, other patients, who spoke at the end of their breaths, were unknowingly making use of another strategy to open locked cords. There are nerve endings in the lungs that detect air volume. When a person exhales most of his air before speaking, these receptors detect what they interpret as the imminent collapse of the lungs, and signal the brain to initiate inspiration. A single pair of muscles at the back of the voice box begins to contract to force the vocal cords apart in preparation for the inflow of air. A person cannot stutter when a pair of muscles is being powerfully driven by the brain to open the vocal cords.

Still others found it easier to speak after first swallowing. During the swallow reflex the vocal cords close tightly to prevent liquids or solid food from entering the lungs, and immediately after the swallow, as part of the same reflex, the cords are opened forcefully so that respiration may resume. These patients had learned that if they started speech at the instant a swallow was completed, they could speak without stuttering.

As for the overt speech struggles—the hesitations, repetitions, prolongations—they, too, seemed to fit this learning model. All were behaviors that were made habitual because they enabled the stutterer to speak, even if he sounded different from everyone else. It works this way: John, struggling to say his name (pulling on the door knob), after a few moments, says it (gets the door open), and the act of saying it (getting the door open) becomes the reward for the struggle (the stutter) which enables him to say it. I now began to suspect that all of the stuttering I observed was a learned response to a common core problem, a spasm of the vocal cords. Here at last, I felt, was the stutter reflex.

The pieces of the puzzle were beginning to come together. From my knowledge of the anatomy and physiology of the speaking apparatus I knew that there are small nerve endings within the vocal cords that detect tension and send this information to the brain. When the tension in the vocal cords builds to a critical locking threshold, these nerve endings issue a particular pattern of impulses. *I now began to understand that it is this particular pattern of nerve impulses reaching the brain that triggers the stutter reflex.*

I asked a colleague who was a specialist in learning psychology if it was possible that so violent and varied a behavior as stuttering could really be learned. His response was to show me a film of learned self-mutilations and to point out that most physically aggressive behaviors are culturally acquired. The struggles I was seeing were mild by comparison. Any behavior that was rewarded could be learned, and the act of speaking which followed the struggle was clearly a sufficient reward to enable the learning of stuttering.

He further pointed out that there was yet another reward commonly present in most human learned behavior and he suspected it to be present for stutterers: anxiety reduction. Anything that could reduce a stutterer's speech anxieties would be rewarded and learned.

I recalled that many stutterers reported that they would often word-substitute rather than stutter. As they spoke they mentally looked ahead so that they could shift the conversation away from feared words or change instantly to a word they could pronounce. The successful avoidance of feared words reduced anxiety, was therefore rewarded, and learned. Word avoidance was as much of a reflex as the stutter itself.

Similarly, many stutterers would consciously try to avoid certain situations that made them nervous—parties, for instance, or interviews, or public speaking of any sort. They learned to go about life selectively—protecting themselves from exposure to stressful situations they knew would cause them to stutter. Of course, in order to successfully avoid these feared words or situations, they had to be constantly vigilant, looking ahead, and so this habit of scanning ahead also became reflexive.

All struggle events, both nonverbal and verbal, were now viewed as learned behaviors—a premise that contradicted many traditional views of stuttering which held that it was a purely psychological condition.

3 *The Stress Connection*

P<small>ROBABLY THE</small> most commonly held notion about stuttering is that it is a psychological problem. It is believed that stutterers have emotional problems or react badly under chronic, excessive stress. As an extreme example, in certain parts of India stutterers are viewed as possessed by demons, and are to be shunned lest the listener catch the contagion, especially if the listener is a child.

There is ample reason to accept a psychological explanation of the cause of stuttering. Stutterers acknowledge that their problem becomes worse under conditions of stress, and report, for example, that when they are alone and under no stress, they have no difficulty speaking fluently.

For years stutterers have been going to psychologists or psychiatrists for treatment. But the published results have not been encouraging: the stuttering has rarely, if ever, improved. The usual explanation offered by the psychotherapist is that the problem is so deep-seated, having most often begun between the ages of two and six, that it would require years of intensive therapy to get to its roots and handle it effectively. This is in spite of the fact that repeated psychological tests have shown stutterers to be totally representative of the normal population.

One stutterer I saw had undergone seventeen years of

psychotherapy at a total cost of approximately $85,000. I remember noting on my evaluation form that this young man was probably the most well-adjusted stutterer I had ever seen.

To this very day, the mythology persists that stuttering is a "psychological problem." Each year books written by so-called experts proclaim this fact, and articles appear frequently in both newspapers and magazines that reinforce the belief. Psychiatrists continue to attempt to treat thousands of stutterers each year using techniques that have long since been proven inadequate.

Freud knew they were inadequate. In one of his early books he wrote, "Whatever the source of stuttering is, it is not amenable to the treatments I have developed. I therefore refuse to attempt to deal with it further."

Nevertheless it was clear to me that while psychological approaches to the treatment of stuttering were ineffective, the role of stress could not be discounted altogether. Somehow stress was effecting the tension at the vocal cords. I discussed the problem with a physiatrist friend who specialized in physical medicine and rehabilitation, and he told me about a study that had been published in 1953. A laboratory had been established in Germany to study the physiology of movement of world-class athletes, with the goal of enhancing athletic ability. As part of this research, the investigators had considered the effects of stress.

The researchers found that the athletes tensed their muscles when stressed, but most interestingly, that they focused tension in certain areas of the body—most commonly the muscles of the shoulder girdle, abdominal wall, lower back, face, and hands. These foci were later termed "targets" and found to be congenital and frequently, but not always, inherited.

There were also less common targets, including the muscles of the vocal cords. The research showed that about

2 percent of the sample studied focused tension at their vocal cords, with a five-to-one ratio of men to women. Subsequent research has revealed that all stutterers come from this 2 percent population and that five times more men stutter than women! This remarkable coincidence revealed to me that the learned stutter reaction has a congenital cause.

The diagram below shows the events associated with stuttering. Some form of stress perceived by the stutterer triggers the locking of the vocal cords; it is an inborn reflex. This in turn triggers stuttering, a learned reflex. So there are two reflexes—one inborn, the other learned. Stutterers are born with the tendency to tense their vocal cords when stressed, and it is the way they learn to handle this tendency that dictates the kind of stuttering they will exhibit.

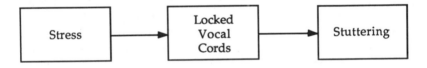

4 *Psychological Triggers of Stuttering*

SINCE STRESS was apparently always required to produce a locking of the vocal cords, I questioned patients about the stresses that provoked their stuttering. I prepared lists of different stresses and asked stuttering patients to indicate which were the most relevant to them. I was looking for common, unifying threads in their observations, and by pooling their responses I was able to identify what seemed to be the most common psychological triggers of stuttering. I call these the stutterer's eight basic stresses.

1. Stressful speaking situations. When I asked stutterers to name the situation in which they found speaking most difficult, the most frequent response was, "On the telephone." Over 80 percent of adult stutterers reported some fear of using the phone. I saw a nineteen-year-old who exemplified this form of stress. A personable young man, he sat in my office and stuttered moderately in response to my questions.

As is customary in my diagnostic evaluations, I asked him to pick up the telephone, call the information operator, and request the telephone number of Macy's department store. He refused. I demanded that he do so, saying that this was an essential part of the evaluation. He pleaded with me not to make him use the telephone. He confessed that he hadn't used it in years and had night-mares about it.

A most unusual situation stress was reported by a priest who was terrified of the thought of speaking in the pulpit. He had stuttered as a child, but thought he had outgrown the habit. After ordination, he had taken a position with a small congregation. A few years later he was given a new post and on his first Sunday entered the church to greet a congregation of eight hundred. The audience size over-whelmed him, his vocal cords locked, and the feedback receptors in his cords triggered a stuttering response that had lain dormant for years.

He began to take tranquilizers, but the dosage required to be effective created undesirable side effects. He decided to leave the church when his physician told him to stop taking the drugs. He approached his bishop with his de-cision, saying that the stuttering was apparently a sign of his "unsuitability." The bishop, a practical man, suggested he try therapy with me first. He did, and four months later was successfully giving sermons again.

2. **Feared words or sounds.** Most people who stutter learn to diligently avoid specific words or sounds they know they will have trouble with. Stutterers can learn to fear any of the sounds, and these fears can change periodically—a person can fear p and t sounds one year and b and k sounds the next. Sometimes a person can lose all fear of specific sounds only to have them return at a later date.

More common are word fears. Almost all adult stutter-ers have some of these, very often fearing only a few spe-cific words. I treated a lawyer who stuttered on only about twenty words. He prepared a list and we practiced them. His problem was treated successfully in a few sessions.

Another patient had a problem saying his first name. He had had it legally changed to a name he had always been able to say easily—and then began to stutter on the new name. When he saw me he was unable to say it. I encouraged him to try and continue to make the attempt in spite of the difficulty he was having. I timed his attempt. The block lasted two minutes and thirty-eight seconds—two minutes and thirty-eight seconds of totally silent and remarkably violent head-thrusting, punctuated only by the occasional drawing of a breath. His convulsions finally concluded in his speaking his name, David.

Another patient reported invariably lying when asked where he grew up because he could not say "Westport." And many patients reported often giving wrong answers in class because they could not say the right ones—and they had to say something. One patient told me he was twenty-eight by saying "the year after twenty-seven." And many patients bemoaned the fact that they were often required to eat what they did not want to eat in restaurants simply because they were unable to say what they wanted.

Word substitution is, at best, awkward, and often frustrating and embarrassing. It is always the result of word or sound stress.

3. Authority figures. Many patients reported difficulty speaking before individuals best described as authority figures. They had trouble talking to the boss or the teacher or when being interviewed. One patient related that when he was stopped by a policeman for speeding he had to take a sobriety test because he was unable to answer the officer's questions. Another reported that throughout school his questions and answers to teachers were written out and read aloud by fellow students.

Virtually all patients report they often stutter only with certain people—for example, with parents. Frequently, parents, noting their children's stuttering at home, request that the school speech therapist treat the problem. But when the child appears before the therapist there is no trace of a stutter. What the therapist is unaware of is that for this child stuttering occurs only in the presence of parental authoritarian stress and that in all other situations it is absent.

One young man I encountered never stuttered with his fiancée but only with her father—not her mother, just her father. Another patient reported that he had never stuttered with a colleague at work until that person was promoted and became his supervisor. In the role of authority figure he became an object capable of provoking stress and consequent stuttering.

4. Uncertainty. Stutterers often have difficulty speaking when they are uncertain about the correct way to pronounce a word or the proper way to behave in an unfamiliar situation—for example, on the first day of a job or when meeting new people.

Nowhere is the stress of uncertainty more manifest than in the difficulties encountered by stutterers attempting to learn a foreign language. There are a number of sources of uncertainty at work here: first, an uncertainty about pronunciation; second, one of vocabulary; and third, grammar. It is no wonder that many patients report stuttering on almost every word in the new language.

5. Fatigue or illness. Stutterers sometimes report more difficulty speaking when tired or ill. Indeed, in the nineteenth century in Europe a school of therapy contended that the primary cause of stuttering was lack of sleep. Patients were often required to sleep as many as fourteen hours a day—as treatment. Some early therapists believed that only a certain part of the body, usually the tongue, was tired and devices were constructed to hold up the "tired" tongue. Generally made of gold or ivory, and worn in the mouth, they usually distracted the individual enough to temporarily stop the stuttering. But after a few days, at most, the stuttering returned with as much intensity as ever.

More recently I encountered several individuals who were treated by a therapist from Russia. His contention was that stuttering was an expression of an overworked speech apparatus, and so he required all his patients to refrain from speaking for six weeks. After this period of total silence they were to start speaking, using single words only for the first several weeks, then using short phrases, and finally full sentences. Needless to say, this technique invariably failed when the first real stress occurred and the vocal cords locked.

Illness is definitely a cause of stress. For example, the country-western singer Mel Tillis started to stutter at the age of three after a bout with malaria, and Winston Churchill's stuttering is attributed to an early severe fall.

6. External factors. This form of stress is also known as "bad news." It is the shock of discovering that you have just been fired or that a relative has a terminal illness or that your car has been stolen. Patients frequently report that external stress figures prominently in their difficulty.

I treated a patient who responded beautifully to my techniques and after a few days of intensive therapy was symptom-free in virtually all situations. He left for his home in Ohio confident of his new skills and equally certain that the continuation of his program would strengthen these new habits and establish them permanently. When he returned, however, he discovered that his house had been burglarized and burned. The external stress was so great that it took him fully six weeks to regain the ability to control his stuttering.

I have seen patients operating in the pressure cooker of the advertising world who, while fluent in most situations after treatment, cannot cope with the external stress of clients continuously contemplating agency changes. I recall seeing an art director whose speech deteriorated further with each subsequent rejection of his artwork by a major client.

7. Speed stress. Probably the most common of all the triggers is what I call speed stress. Speed stress is responsible for the onset of most stuttering in children. It is the product of speaking too rapidly.

Almost all stutterers suffer from speed stress to some degree. For very young children, speed stress is often the sole trigger of stuttering. When they speak slowly, these children become fluent. Adults, on the other hand, have more complicated stresses, and thus for most adults slow speaking does not result in immediate fluency.

Most adult stutterers are not aware of speaking too rapidly. Indeed, when I measured the average number of words they spoke per minute, when fluent, it was well within normal limits—approximately 130 words per minute. When we measured the speed of the first word in a sentence, however, it was found to be as much as four times faster than average. Instead of beginning speech in a slow and leisurely manner, stutterers attack their words.

One patient, who invariably stuttered on the first word of each sentence, indicated that the reason he spoke so quickly was that he "wanted to get away from the scene of the crime as quickly as possible." What he did not realize, of course, was that this desire was resulting in speed stress and thereby helping to create the very block he was seeking to escape.

8. Base-level stress. There are sixteen muscles in and around the vocal cords, and by putting an electrode on any one of them one could easily record the tension developed within. This tension is always present, but its magnitude can fluctuate widely. The fluctuation occurs in response to two major influences.

The first are brain hormones—which, through their chemical effects on certain cerebral centers, have the capability of increasing muscle tension dramatically. When patients report their speech has suddenly worsened, and can find no obvious reason for it, the usual explanation is an increased production of these hormones.

The second source of tension are persistent, long-standing subconscious conflicts which become exacerbated by a change in one's life circumstances. It may be a new job, with a boss whose demeanor parallels a parent's—setting off a sequence of underlying emotional reactions which go unrecognized but wreak havoc with speech. Or perhaps it's a spouse's decision to make a major life change, which subtly upsets the well-defined structure of the relationship, provoking anxiety and subsequent negative effects upon speech—despite the fact that both parties consciously acknowledge the absolute desirability of the change.

When both factors are present simultaneously and are in combination with any of the other seven stresses, the total tension on the vocal cords can mount to the point where the patient is virtually incapable of speaking. This is seen often in young children, whose base-level stress has been shown to vary widely over time. Parents are particularly frustrated by this and report that their child can often go for weeks without stuttering only to find that overnight the dysfluencies return with full force. Many such children are brought to my office during one of their fluent periods. The parents are quick to assure me that their child stutters and sometimes violently, and in a sense apologize for their child's lack of difficulty. They almost invariably say that they are unable to account for these fluctuations and their guilt is assuaged when base-level stress is explained to them.

5 Four Types of Stuttering

Fʀᴏᴍ ᴀ ᴄᴀʀᴇꜰᴜʟ examination of a large number of patients, we identified four types of stuttering, which we called Types 1 through 4. Type 1 refers to the process shown in the diagram below. The horizontal line indicates time moving forward from left to right; the time period is several seconds. The three dots on the line indicate the three steps of the stutter reflex. Stress leads to a locking of the vocal cords, which shortly precedes the stutter, which *coincides in time with speech.*

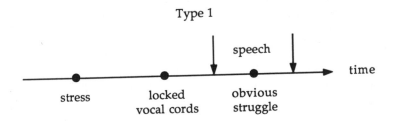

Type 1 is considered the most common form of stuttering. The struggle with speech consists of hesitations, and repetitions and prolongations of sounds, syllables, or words. When the average nonstuttering individual thinks of stuttering, it is Type 1 he has in mind.

In Type 2 stuttering, stress again leads to the locking of the vocal cords which reflexively triggers a struggle, but in this instance the struggle is not part of speech but *precedes* it. The struggling may be violent but the stutterer has elected to delay speech until after the struggle—so the speech, when it occurs, is fluent.

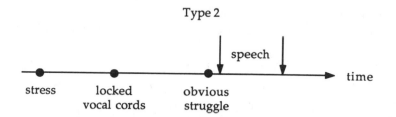

Type 2

stress   locked   obvious
              vocal cords   struggle

speech

time

Type 2 stutterers are fascinating to observe as they speak on the telephone. Their head may be thrust back in some violent gesture, their jaw may shake, eyes clench, hands thrust—while the person at the other end hears nothing, just a pause followed by normal-sounding speech.

I once treated such a stutterer in England. The day before treatment, I had arranged to meet him at a small airport just outside of London. He was a pilot and had offered a bird's-eye view of the city and surrounding countryside.

Because he was a Type 2 stutterer, his speech on the radio to the tower sounded normal, but the struggle taking place in the cockpit as we taxied to the runway suggested I was about to have a bumpy ride. And indeed it was, for his prespeech struggles involved his entire body, including both arms and legs. Each sentence that emerged fluently was preceded by a brief but hair-raising form of aerial aerobatics that left me exhausted and air-sick at the end of the flight.

We had arranged that he would drive me back to London. The trip took about an hour and I recall speaking

almost incessantly, since whenever he spoke, the car
lurched.

The Type 2 stutterer demonstrates that the struggle to
release the vocal-cord spasm is clearly independent of
speech. The fact that for most stutterers the struggle appears in the speech (Type 1) is simply an expression of
their inability to wait and complete their struggles before
starting to speak.

In Type 3 stuttering, stress once again provokes the lock-

Type 3

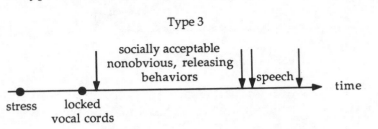

ing of the vocal cords, but here the stutterer elects not to
struggle but rather to pause and wait for the locked cords
to release. This may be accomplished by several means: he
may distract himself in some appropriate manner, he may
passively wait for his stress to drop, he may quietly inhale
to open his vocal cords, or he may swallow to achieve the
same end. One patient I treated would cough gently during such pauses to blow his vocal cords apart.

Another patient would pause, smile, and look up at the
ceiling as if deep in thought before responding. If one
looked closely at his Adam's apple, however, one observed that it bobbed up and down very rapidly during
these "reflective" pauses. The patient was actually engaged in a series of very rapid swallows to open his vocal
cords. If a single swallow was sufficient the pause would
be brief. But if his cords locked again too quickly, it might
be necessary to swallow two, three, or four times in quick
succession to speak. Beneath the smile and apparent
thoughtfulness lay a violent, hidden, and single-minded

struggle to deal with a spasm that blocked both breathing and speech.

Finally, in Type 4 stuttering the stuttering chain is aborted before it starts. The stutterer has made a conscious habit of scanning ahead for "trouble," and when he sees it avoids the situation altogether.

Type 4

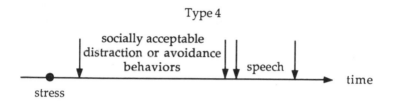

Type 4 stuttering is referred to as hidden or "closet" stuttering and is discussed more fully in the next chapter. Twenty percent of all patients seen at the National Center for Stuttering fit this category. These patients avoid threatening words, sounds, and speaking situations. No one knows they stutter, but the price they pay for their fluency is constant vigilance.

Type 1 stuttering is the "typical" form, seen most often in stutterers. The struggles are part of speech. Type 2 stuttering, though less frequent, is also recognized as stuttering even though the speech is unimpaired. Type 3 and Type 4 stuttering are socially acceptable; they are generally not recognized as forms of stuttering. Stutterers in these two categories rarely seek professional help even though these forms of the disorder often take a considerable emotional toll.

As I examined more and more adult stutterers, I began to notice different combinations of the four types. For example, a patient might struggle with the pronunciation of her name, substitute one word for another while describing her occupation, and cough to release her vocal cords before describing an experience. I discovered that a mixture of types within patients was the rule rather than the exception. There were, of course, "pure" types—mostly Type 1 and 2—and clinicians saw them on occasion. Types 3 and 4 were rarely seen in therapy, not because they did not exist in substantial numbers, but rather because they did not seek assistance.

6 *Closet Stutterers*

MY WORK with stutterers confirmed the often-noted research finding that stutterers as a group are above average in intelligence. One manifestation of this intelligence is that they quickly learn to scan for words they fear and to either shift the conversation or substitute synonyms. All stutterers do this to some extent, but some become so adroit at it that they appear to stop stuttering altogether. I have labeled these "closet stutterers," and they constitute approximately 20 percent of all patients seen for treatment.

While any profile of stutterers shows that approximately five times as many men have this problem as women, the statistics for closet stutterers are reversed. In the study reported in the appendix of this book, 87 of the patients were closet stutterers—62 females and 25 males, or a ratio of two and a half to one favoring females. It appears that women elect to hide stuttering more often than men.

Winston Churchill was a closet stutterer and his vast vocabulary was in large measure due to the fact that he was continually word-substituting. Closet stutterers are walking thesauruses; they do crossword puzzles in ink. And since they don't stutter, they function well in society.

I recall evaluating a closet stutterer and then later communicating with him by mail. His wife called to say that she had received the letter and wondered what it was all about since in their nineteen years of marriage her husband had never stuttered. I explained to her that he was a closet stutterer and that he avoided certain words, sounds, and speaking situations. There was a long pause and then a torrent of questions: "Do you think that's why he has me make the phone calls, and why I always wind up ordering in restaurants, and why he never speaks up at PTA meetings?" As she asked these questions, which were in a sense rhetorical, I could hear that she was beginning to understand something she had never known about her husband. I suggested she speak with him about his problem since I felt that if he was to undergo successful treatment, her support would be invaluable.

Closet stutterers report they are exhausted at the end of the day. There is no such thing as an idle conversation; they are always "on," hunting, substituting, avoiding. In a sense they are more stressed than the overt stutterer, because for the latter, everyone knows, "it all hangs out." But if no one knows, then one must maintain a constant vigilance, and this is always fatiguing.

Closet stutterers report that in an effort to hide their stuttering they frequently say things that are inappropriate, foolish, or nonsensical. They also often leave sentences hanging in the hope that the listener will fill in the missing (difficult) words.

I recall treating a hairdresser named Pierre who spoke with a thick French accent. As part of my evaluation, I asked him where he was born and he responded, "Brooklyn." Thinking that he had been raised in France, I asked him where he had gone to school. And again he responded, "Brooklyn." "So your accent is phony?" I said. "Yup," he answered without a trace of an accent. He then recounted his discovery that if he spoke in this manner he tended not to stutter, and people would forgive him for the fractured English that his word substitution required. Also, if he couldn't say a particular word, such as "comb," he could easily point to the comb and say, "How you say in English?" This strategy had worked well for him until his brother-in-law suggested that he take a job in his insurance agency. He wanted the position and so now sought treatment.

Closet stutterers will go to inordinate extents to hide their difficulty. I evaluated a man who was a judge in a state supreme court in New England. He had been a closet stutterer for over thirty years, and although his word-substitution habits had sometimes resulted in rather unusual language, he was so good at it that, in a sense, it added to his speaking charisma.

He controlled his stress by taking a moderate dose of Valium each day, and had done so for over fifteen years. While on a Caribbean cruise with his wife, he decided to forgo the Valium and within a day began to have seizures—the sign of Valium dependency. He immediately went back on the drug.

He was a respected member of his community and much admired for his legal expertise. It was no surprise when he was asked to take a federal district judgeship. But he refused the offer and no one knew why. He gave some excuse about liking the kind of work he was doing, when everyone knew the federal position was a real prize.

He came to see me for two reasons. First, he wanted to be able to gradually reduce his Valium intake, and this he felt could only be accomplished if he eliminated the stresses associated with being a closet stutterer. Second, he knew he wouldn't be able to advance in his profession unless he overcame his affliction. This turned out to be the real reason for his refusal of the federal district judgeship: on the state court he was allowed to paraphrase the charge to the jury, whereas on the federal court he would have had to read it word-for-word, and couldn't substitute. Thus he obviously couldn't take the position.

He was now confiding this for the first time, and the

apparent release of tension associated with this confession reduced his stress level considerably. I did not treat him immediately; he was at first unwilling to substitute my technique for his well-established avoidance behaviors. But a year later, when he was again offered a position he wanted, he presented himself for treatment and was successful.

Closet stutterers make more rapid progress in treatment than overt stutterers because they have less to accomplish—they already function well in society and are not viewed by themselves or their peers as handicapped. Their self-esteem and socialization skills tend to be good, and when they stop word-substituting they usually can make a seamless transition into their everyday activities. Overt stutterers, on the other hand, have a direct and negative effect upon their environment and suffer as a result. Their socialization skills tend to be poor and when they no longer stutter they must learn entirely new skills for interacting with others. As one patient said to me, "Dr. Schwartz, now that I don't stutter, what do I say to people, what do I talk about?"

I often tell closet stutterers: "If you stutter openly and you stop, it is a gift to the world because the world is no longer required to see and hear you stutter—and a gift to yourself because you know you are free of the affliction. But when you are a closet stutterer, it is a gift just to yourself; you can't expect society to know or care or be interested in your hidden problem. The gift, of course, is this incredible sense of freedom to be able to say whatever you want to say, wherever you want to say it, whenever you want to say it—without fear."

7 Primary Versus Secondary Stuttering

Our consideration of the speech symptoms of stuttering would be incomplete without noting the difference between the beginning and advanced forms of the disorder. They have been labeled primary and secondary stuttering, and have traditionally been defined in terms of the forcefulness and location of the struggles. The primary stutterer is said to show effortless repetitions only at the beginnings of sentences, and the secondary stutterer struggles forcefully anywhere in the sentence.

My examination of patients led me to conclude that the force distinction was erroneous. For example, 20 percent of patients are hidden or "closet" stutterers, as noted previously. They never struggle openly but rather look ahead for difficult sounds, words, and situations and avoid them. No one knows they stutter; their overt struggle symptoms are less than mild—they are nonexistent. I therefore developed the following three diagnostic questions which have been shown to yield far more useful information.

1. When you speak, do you sometimes look ahead for difficult words and try to substitute one word for another?

2. Can you usually tell when you are going to stutter just before it happens?
3. Do you stutter when you talk to yourself out loud alone?

A primary stutterer will answer no to all three questions. Indeed, for the very young child, the questions may not make sense, and this lack of understanding is a positive sign that the child has no anticipatory stress. Children who respond this way will invariably show repetitions or hesitations only at the beginnings of sentences. The behaviors may, however, be forceful.

The secondary stutterer will usually say yes to the first two questions and no to the last. If he responds yes to the last question, it is an indication that his overall stress is high. The secondary stutterer usually exhibits strong struggle behaviors which can occur anywhere in the sentence.

Using the severity of the struggle as the major distinction between primary and secondary stuttering is, as I have indicated, invalid. Rather, the distinction has to be the presence or absence of *anticipatory stress*. Does the patient see the sounds, words, or fearful speaking situations approaching? If the answer is no, the patient is a primary stutterer. If yes, he is a secondary stutterer—he scans ahead for "trouble." Generally most children under seven are primary stutterers, while most over the age of ten are secondary. And during the three-year interval between, there is a period of transitional stuttering.

During this transitional period, a child may report fear of speaking in certain situations, while at the same time he will have no recognition of the words or sounds which cause him difficulty. Also during this period, some children will report that they can see some of the feared words coming but that others are a surprise. The average eight-year-old will understand the following line of questioning:

"Sometimes you have trouble with your speech, don't you? When you have trouble, do you know what words you are going to have trouble with—can you see the hard words coming?" The child may respond, "Sometimes." This is followed with the question, "You mean sometimes you can tell and sometimes it's a surprise—is that right?" Usually the child will say yes and the next question is, "Is it mostly a surprise or mostly you can tell?"

If the child says it's mostly a surprise we can be fairly certain he is at the beginning of the transitional period. But if he reports that mostly he can tell, we must then view him as an adult stutterer and treat him accordingly.

While it is generally correct to say that most children under the age of seven are primary stutterers and those over the age of ten are secondary, it is clear there are many exceptions to this rule. I have seen precocious five-year-olds with well-established sound, word, and situation fears coupled with strong struggle behaviors and word substitutions. And I have also seen teenagers with no word or sound anticipations and only minor effortless repetitions at the beginnings of sentences.

It is important to be able to recognize the presence or absence of anticipatory stress in a stutterer because it directly relates to the expected outcome of therapy. A child with no word or sound fears is unaware of his difficulty and thus does not suffer greatly. He is not motivated to work on his problem, and so the likelihood of recovery is not nearly so good. The secondary stutterer, on the other hand, lives in continuous anticipatory dread of feared words and sounds, and is in considerable emotional pain, and thus is highly motivated to improve.

I attempted to treat several children who were clearly either primary or beginning transitional stutterers. In each instance, the child learned the techniques for stopping stuttering and upon returning home began practicing with a parent. In each instance, the technique produced complete fluency, but the child had no interest in continuing with the prescribed exercises.

The parents found themselves badgering the child and an initial willingness to work disintegrated. They would call to express frustration and I would respond by altering the mix of exercises. But this, too, soon lost its power to sustain interest.

We would then use a reward system in which the child would be given a gold star for a correct sequence of performances. At a later time these could be redeemed for a prize. The reward system worked well for some but for others it, too, failed to sustain.

I soon realized that direct therapy with primary stutterers would rarely be successful, and I decided not to take on these children as patients. But some can be helped, and later in this book I will present a series of indirect approaches that have proven successful with a large number of primary stutterers.

My case records show several examples of children worked with unsuccessfully as primary stutterers who demonstrated a successful outcome five years later after they had become secondary. In a sense it is very much like pneumonia: you may not be able to treat them when they have a cold, but you can when they have pneumonia.

Part II

TREATMENT

8 *Attempts at Correction*

THE RANGE of treatments for stuttering has been extensive. Hundreds of books and thousands of articles have been published on the subject in the last half century. Certain techniques occur repeatedly in the literature because they have been partially successful; others, unfortunately, have been much less so. Anyone concerned with stuttering needs to know about the strengths and weaknesses of the various therapies available.

Relaxation therapies
These have been by far the most prevalent approaches to the treatment of stuttering. There are several varieties of relaxation therapy, but in all of them the aim is to reduce muscle tensions throughout the body, and thus elude the stutter reflex. In one approach, patients are encouraged to start by focusing on a specific muscle group (usually the toes), contract it maximally to heighten awareness of the tension, and then relax it as much as possible. Each muscle group is addressed separately until the entire body is relaxed. This procedure, known as *progressive relaxation,* was first described in 1923 by Edmund Jacobson, and has been employed frequently for the treatment of stuttering. The reported results indicate improvement but never total success in eliminating the problem.

Another type of relaxation involves yoga-derived *stretching exercises.* These involve twisting, rotating, and bending the torso, and increasing the flexibility of the spine. Performed slowly and in a deeply meditative state, these exercises gradually bring their practitioners a more tranquil demeanor—the result again being improvement, but not total arrestment.

In *guided imagery*, patients are trained to imagine a restful scene or tranquil activity and then encouraged to dwell on the image periodically throughout the day. This technique produces substantial relaxation in some patients, again with attendant improvements in speech.

Finally, there are the *biofeedback* approaches. Electrodes are attached to various muscles (usually on the neck) and the degrees of tension developed during speech are registered on a meter. Patients are trained to lower tension by focusing on the meter as they attempt to make the level decrease. Unfortunately, the findings with biofeedback have been disappointing, since following treatment the stuttering rarely improves.

In summary, it appears that relaxation approaches tend to improve or reduce stuttering, but do not stop it. They simply do not subtract enough tension from the vocal cords.

Deep breathing exercises

It is felt that breathing deeply before speaking stops stuttering. Based on this premise, some therapies teach a variety of deep breathing exercises. A few of these techniques stress breathing from the diaphragm, while others stress the rib cage. Some therapists talk about the importance of nasal breathing; others, oral. The justification for the exercises is the oft-noted observation that the breathing patterns of stutterers are disturbed. Unfortunately, most of the experimental studies have shown no improvement.

Speaking exercises

Some therapies try to tackle the problem of stuttering directly by teaching a new way of speaking altogether—like a new language. For example, some therapists have advocated using speech timed to the rhythm of a metronome, while others have suggested using what is best described as a singsong voice. Some require their patients to speak softly; others require them to shout. Still others have suggested that the pitch be raised, while just as many are equally emphatic that pitch must be lowered. Other suggestions to patients have included speaking with a foreign accent, speaking as they inhale, hardly moving the mouth while speaking, and whispering.

A survey of the outcome of these often contradictory approaches shows them to be largely ineffective. This is not to suggest that new ways of speaking do not produce fluency—on the contrary, they often do. But they are ineffective as a form of therapy because patients reject them. They are perceived as alien; they are not normal. Patients may not like stuttering but at least they are used to it. They are not used to talking in a manner which they and others perceive as strange.

For example, it is known that every stutterer in the world will be fluent if he sings. But show me a stutterer who is willing to break into song every time he wants to communicate. It is just not acceptable. The country-western singer Mel Tillis has made a career of juxtaposing a totally fluent singing voice against the difficulty he experiences whenever he tries to speak. He does this in a humorous vein and has his audience laughing along with him at the incongruity.

It has also been well documented that one can stop stuttering by speaking slowly. Proponents of this approach are known as the *controlled rate group*. These therapists claim the reason slow speech helps stuttering is that it allows the brain time to compensate for the presumed but unspecified incoordination among the respiratory, vocal cord, and articulatory mechanisms.

One method commonly employed for slowing speech is called *delayed auditory feedback*. Patients speak into a microphone attached to a tiny computer which records, delays, and sends amplified speech to earphones. The patient hears his speech delayed by approximately two-tenths of a second. Speaking under such conditions is difficult; one tries continuously to adjust to or compensate for the delay.

It turns out that the only successful way to compensate is to slow the rate of speaking. While the slowing reduces or even eliminates stuttering, the price one pays, apart from the obvious slowness of the speech, is the obtrusiveness of having to speak into a microphone, wear a computer, and have earphones on all the time.

In another method a tiny electronic metronome is inserted behind the ear. The speed of the metronome can be adjusted as the person speaks, so he is required to time his syllables to the rate he hears in his ear. Providing the beat is slow enough, this *syllable-timed speech*, as it is called, produces fluency. But again, the price paid is unnatural-sounding speech and dependency on an electronic device.

Proponents counter by saying that patients can gradually increase the speed of the metronome, and when it is sufficiently rapid, the speech sounds normal and the patient can then discard it. The experience of stutterers, however, shows that as the rate is increased, stuttering reappears.

Punishment

Punishment has a long history in the treatment of stuttering. For example, electric shocks have been and continue to be employed to create unpleasant stimuli. No one likes a shock, however mild it may be, and a patient will do anything to avoid one.

But the psychology of learning tells us that people learn because they are rewarded, and a shock is punishment, something to be avoided. Patients will do whatever is necessary to avoid getting shocked, whether it means changing the pitch of their voice, swallowing, coughing, speaking slowly, or sounding as unnatural as they can. But this does not mean that they *learn* these techniques.

As soon as the shock is removed they quickly revert to stuttering.

Another form of punishment used with stutterers was carbon dioxide treatment. Carbon dioxide has been used to treat depression and other mental problems; it was often used as a substitute for electroconvulsive shock therapy. Recently, a patient in her early sixties reported being forced to breath CO_2 as a child. She recalled being taken every morning by her father to a doctor who would administer pure CO_2 through a face mask. After two breaths she would pass out and, when revived, be driven to school. This went on for a year and a half without any positive effect on her speech, and the memory of this daily torture has remained etched in her mind for over half a century.

Surgery, while not necessarily punishment, had the same effect. Surgical approaches were employed in Europe in the middle of the nineteenth century and still continue today, albeit to a much lesser extent. For example, if a stutterer lived in Germany in 1842 there was a good likelihood that he would have had a portion or all of his tongue removed. (Bear in mind that this was before the advent of anesthesia!) Surgeons pursued this course for almost fifteen years before they decided it was ineffective.

Even today, one sees well-meaning physicians suggesting that the cause of stuttering is tongue-tie and that the problem can be cured simply by snipping the small piece of tissue they feel tethers the tongue to the floor of the mouth. Unfortunately, there is no evidence that this approach has any positive effects upon speech whatsoever, and one can only hope that the practice will cease.

Drugs

The last approach to the treatment of stutterers is the administration of drugs. These fall into three basic categories. The first is the anticonvulsants. Neurologists consider the violent struggle behaviors associated with stuttering to be a form of convulsive seizure. But lacking training in learning psychology, they fail to understand that such struggles are learned. The medical literature is filled with published reports of the merits of one anticonvulsant drug over another for the treatment of stuttering. The fact that the vast majority of patients do not stop stuttering and that the side effects of the drugs are often serious does not seem to dissuade neurologists from pursuing this treatment.

The second class of drugs used to treat stuttering is the tranquilizers. There are a number of these and many have been proven useful in reducing overall stress. But again, they do not completely eliminate the problem, and their side effects can be substantial. Recently tested are a new family of tranquilizers called beta-blockers. These show promise and further research is under way.

The third group comprises the muscle relaxants. If tension is the ultimate source of stuttering, it makes good sense to investigate any approach that reduces tension. However, it appears that the amount of any drug necessary to reduce vocal-cord tension is so great that the side effects are invariably unpleasant and unsafe.

CLEARLY THERE has been great interest in developing methods for treating stuttering. Most treatments bring at least some relief to a significant percentage of stutterers. But none solve the problem completely, and that ultimately creates their downfall. It's very much like cancer. You remove 90 percent of the cancer and the other 10 percent does you in. Unless you can eliminate all of the stuttering, the residual will eventually create the inevitable relapse.

9 *The Passive Airflow Technique*

AFTER I discovered the physical basis of stuttering and established the role stress plays, I began to consider the implications that this new model of stuttering would have on treatment. Clearly, any therapy would have to address both the actual physical response—the locking of the vocal cords—and the psychological triggers associated with it.

I began talking to so-called "recovered" stutterers, hoping to gain some insight into the interaction between these two components of stuttering. I actually ran an ad in a local newspaper, and offered twenty dollars for the privilege of an interview.

The interviews with 42 "recovered" stutterers showed some to be speaking a bit more slowly than usual, though not remarkably so. I also found that eleven of them exhibited tiny airflows in their speech. Using a metal mirror against the lips to record condensation, I could visually detect a small amount of air coming from their mouths just before they spoke. It was as if they preceded each sentence with a tiny, inaudible sigh.

The more I thought about this, the more intrigued I became. What were these tiny airflows? What function did they serve? I never saw them in the speech of stutterers, nor in the speech of normal speakers with no history of stuttering. Why, then, in this group?

I remember sitting in my office mimicking the flows. And then it hit me: the answer was in the flow. The flow was being used to ensure an opening of the vocal cords prior to speaking. The flow was passive, never pushed, and its sigh-like quality appeared to keep the cords apart and relaxed.

I could now explain the bizarre behavior of a patient whom I had seen earlier who stated that he never stuttered when he smoked. When I asked him to demonstrate, he lit a cigarette, inhaled, let out some of the smoke, and began to speak. The stuttering disappeared.

When I asked him why he thought it helped, he said it relaxed him. I passed it off as a form of psychological distraction. Little did I suspect at that time that the answer to the problem was to be seen in the smoke being blown past my face.

Later, through my reading, I was to discover that the vocal cords are controlled by the breathing centers of the brain. During normal, quiet respiration they open slightly just before inhalation, then close slightly as the airflow is reversed and exhalation begins.

The opening of the vocal cords has been shown to be an active process, the result of the contraction of a single pair of muscles located at the rear of the voice box. The exhalation phase, on the other hand, is passive, the inward movement of the vocal cords occurring as the muscles relax. Research has shown that the most relaxed state of the vocal cords occurs during this expiratory phase of normal, quiet respiration.

In other research, electrodes have been placed on the vocal cords to study the tension patterns associated with speech. The tensions in the vocal cords before speech have also been studied. The research shows that the average person starts to tense his vocal cords between one-third second and one-half second before he speaks.

This fraction of a second before speech begins appears to be critical because it is the time during which the vocal cords can and often do lock. I had observed this earlier in my ultrasonic scans of the vocal cords in stutterers. I reasoned that if I could help stutterers reduce these prespeech vocal-cord tensions they would stand an excellent chance of keeping their cords from locking and thus stopping stuttering.

The trick, then, was to somehow learn to exhale just before speaking as if one were *not going to speak at all but were simply quietly breathing.* The brain had to be fooled into believing that the speaker was simply taking another breath. If the brain was fooled, it would develop no prespeech tensions on the cords.

I began to experiment with an airflow technique. I started by asking a stutterer to produce a long, audible, relaxed sigh. I then asked him to sigh once again, and when halfway through to say a one-syllable word. The stuttering stopped. I increased the number of one-syllable words spoken on a breath. Again, no stuttering.

I was amazed. It seemed so simple. But day after day my results were confirmed—the patient's speech continued to be fluent. My spirits began to rise. I kept wondering how long it would be before the inevitable relapse, but it did not occur, and I decided to proceed to the next step. I asked the patient to make the flows inaudible. He did so immediately, explaining that he had practiced this at home since he did not care to go about sounding "like a breathy pervert." His speech was now totally acceptable, and he remained fluent.

Here, I thought, was a technique that was the essence of simplicity. It focused specifically upon what I had theorized to be the cause of stuttering. The passive airflow kept the vocal cords apart and relaxed prior to speech and deprived the brain of the signals necessary to trigger the stutter reflex.

But for other patients, the immediacy of the result belied

a subsequent period of difficulty. Although they used the airflow continuously, they still stuttered at times. What was wrong?

I recorded examples of these occurrences of stuttering from a number of patients and, after listening to them, found four mistakes which seemed to provoke the reappearance of stuttering. I called them *misuses of airflow*, and all patients were subsequently given instructions to alert them to these mistakes so they might avoid them at all times.

1. Pushing the flow. Under conditions of stress, patients tended to push or force the flow, which frequently led to a locking of the vocal cords and a subsequent stutter. They were reminded that the flow had to be absolutely passive, that a pushed flow would sooner or later be interpreted by the brain as an *h*, and that the brain would then "think" that all sentences began with an *h* and the stuttering would reappear.

2. Failure of transition. Another source of difficulty was the lack of a smooth flow into the first sound of the first word. *The flow appeared short, with a pause between the end of the flow and the beginning of speech.* It appeared as if the patient were catching his breath—as if, perhaps, to initiate an inhalation. The pause provided the time necessary for the cords to lock. I told patients, "The airflow is your lifeline to fluency; follow it directly into the word."

3. Failure of intent. Patients are often so preoccupied with the upcoming first sound that their mouths form the position for that sound during the final instants of airflow. Thus the airflow is affected by the anticipated sound, and one of the effects of such anticipation is always a tensing of the vocal cords—which often leads to a stutter. Patients are reminded that the object of the airflow is to fool the brain into believing that they are just simply taking another breath. If they start to form the first sound of the first word before they say it, the brain is not fooled.

4. Holding the flow. In an effort to time their flows, patients often inhale and hold the air by closing their vocal cords, then start the airflow at the appropriate time by releasing their cords. If they attempt to do this under stress, the hold is often transformed into a lock and they stutter.

Patients were instructed never to hold the flow but to keep the air in continuous movement, that is, to inhale smoothly and then just as smoothly reverse the flow and exhale; there was never to be a stoppage of the flow at any point.

With these cautions in mind my patients were now responding well. The airflow technique, when practiced properly, brought substantial improvement. But occasionally, stuttering blocks still occurred. Despite the use of seemingly perfect airflows, some patients continued to experience difficulty.

Reexamining these patients, I would, for example, hear a young man use perfect airflow into a *t* and then stutter. I tape-recorded a number of instances of these unexplainable blocks and played them over and over.

As I was listening to them at home one evening, wondering if I would ever find a solution, my wife entered the room and said, "You know, those people speak awfully fast."

And then I realized the obvious: these people were speed-stressing themselves. If a patient was afraid of a sound, even though he used perfect airflow he would rush through the word which contained the sound. As a result of this rushed word, the brain would tense the vocal-cord muscles, anticipating rapid speech to follow. It's much the same process as when a sprinter tenses his leg muscles a split second before starting a 100-yard dash. But while tensed leg muscles in a sprinter give him a clear advantage, tensed vocal cord muscles in a stutterer obstruct his airflow and result in a stutter.

In a sense, then, getting set to speak should be the same as getting set to run a twenty-six-mile marathon. The marathoner doesn't need the high initial acceleration of a sprinter, and if we measure the tension in his leg muscles a split second before the race, we find considerably less of it.

If our goal with stutterers is to subtract as much tension as possible from the vocal cords prior to the start of speech, a slow start is critical. Indeed, when I forced patients to say the first word slowly, the stuttering was averted.

I have found the combination of the passive airflow and the slowed first word to constitute a powerful defense against stuttering, and it is what I have come to call *perfect technique*. With perfect technique it is impossible to stutter. I began to inform patients of this very important fact. I arranged multiple-stress speaking situations so that each patient could see the truth of this dictum firsthand. Patients invariably felt much less anxiety and stress, and the beneficial effect of their successful performance was powerful and obvious. Here, for the first time, was a clear-cut prescription for fluency.

I now felt sufficiently well informed about the stutter response to be able to experiment with different methods of treatment.

10 *The Workshop*

ORIGINALLY I worked with patients on a one-to-one basis, but about twelve years ago I began to experiment working with them in pairs, and I have found performance in the paired situation to be clearly superior. The presence of another patient increased stress by making the performance slightly public and introducing an element of competition.

Initially, I matched patients according to age and sex. But I found no differences when I paired dissimilar individuals. This held true for both the type and the severity of stuttering.

I then began to experiment with larger groups—first three people, then six, twelve, and so on. Again, no difference could be seen for the variable of number of participants, except, of course, that as the number grew larger, the amount of time necessary to achieve the desired therapeutic goals lengthened. I finally settled on fifteen patients as the maximum I would treat together, and the length of each treatment session increased from one hour to three hours and then to an entire day. I found that the group structure coupled with a full day gave each patient ample opportunity to participate during the session, and maintained just enough stress that speaking was a challenge but not an impossibility. Patients learned from one another's mistakes, and each time a patient spoke it was, by definition, public speaking.

After much trial and error, here is the treatment format that we found to be most effective, and that we now use in our workshops at the National Center for Stuttering.

Breathing

We start by teaching patients to breathe passively from their mouths. I ask them to imagine themselves with a cold, with their noses stuffed and able only to breathe from the mouth. I reinforce this by saying that they carry with them at all times the perfect model of the breath. It is the calm breathing they engage in when they are sitting quietly, doing nothing—except now it's through the mouth. I continue to talk to them and watch their mouths, chests, and abdominal walls for signs of passive outflows of air.

Once passive airflows from the mouth are established, we move on to using them before monosyllables and then multisyllables. At this point we introduce several feedback techniques that have been developed for monitoring airflow. By enabling patients to hear their own breathing patterns, these devices help them recognize the particular sound quality of a totally passive airflow. This quality of sound is called *flutter*, and differs from person to person since everyone's respiratory system is shaped differently. Every patient must learn to recognize his own characteristic flutter pattern. For some this takes no time at all; for others it takes more practice—but whatever the time involved, no progress can be made in airflow treatment without first attaining a consistent flutter.

The simplest, and probably the most effective feedback technique involves a piece of rubber tubing about a foot long. One end of the tubing is placed directly in front of the speaker's lips and the other is placed in his ear. Thus the patient can listen to his breathing.

Another common feedback device is a tape recorder. The patient breathes into a special microphone which is capable of picking up minute airflows from the mouth. These flows are tape-recorded and played back for evaluation. The patient must learn to recognize his flutter on the tape recorder.

The presence of flutter indicates a totally passive airflow. But when the airflow is no longer passive, flutter is replaced by one of two classes of breathing sounds: pushed or squeezed flows. A pushed flow indicates that the patient is actively aiding the outflow of air, while a squeezed airflow is produced when the vocal cords are already locked and the patient is forcing the air between them. During workshops, pushed and squeezed flows are recorded and played back for training purposes. Much time is spent practicing this extremely basic and critical phase of the program, since pushed and squeezed flows invariably lead to stuttering and are to be avoided at all costs.

When flutter before single words is produced consistently, we proceed to the production of flutter before short phrases and then before short sentences. We teach two rules to deal with the problem of the quick start. The first rule applies when a phrase or sentence begins with a one-syllable word: "When a sentence or phrase begins with a one-syllable word, we are to put a comma, a mental pause, between the first word and the rest of the sentence." The second rule relates to phrases or sentences beginning with a multisyllable word: "When the first word is a multisyllable, we must say each syllable with equal slowing, much as if it were spoken to the rhythm of a slow me-tro-nome."

All patients are given special lists of phrases and sentences to practice. All practice is performed using the rubber tube to monitor for the passive outflow of air and the slowed first word. In addition, periodic samples are recorded on a cassette and played back for evaluation.

At the end of the first treatment session I ask each patient to stand in front of the group and give a short speech. A few hours earlier, the thought of such an activity would have been an impossibility; now they are speaking perfectly—without a trace of a stutter.

As each person's turn comes to speak, the others are required to subvocally practice with the patient. In this way, practice is fairly continuous. In addition, I continuously scan the room observing these subvocal practices to make certain that they are done correctly. If I see a misuse of airflow or a failure to slow the first word, I note it publicly and emphatically, thereby stressing the extreme importance of powerfully attending to technique.

Contract

I developed a one-minute exercise I called "Contract" to deal with the problem of attending to technique. After patients demonstrate both an understanding and ability to produce a passive airflow together with a slowed first word, they are required to recite a string of unrelated sentences out loud for one minute in front of an audience. Unrelated sentences are chosen initially because related ones would form a context which might distract the patient's attention from his fledgling technique. Each sentence must be perfect, and if the speaker happens to stutter, he is required to pay a dollar for every block. My typical comment in announcing this is, "Now that you have shown that you can control your stuttering you must pay for the privilege of inflicting your struggle behavior on the world around you." Initially, Contract is done for one minute a day. Later the duration is increased.

We have found that patients' attention to technique while under Contract is outstanding. The slightest tendency for the mind to wander is effectively canceled by the knowledge that if they stutter they have to pay up. All monies collected during Contract are usually given to the youngest individual at the workshop, who has been elected to buy me lunch. Alas, I often can't even raise enough money for dessert.

I recall treating a young man from Houston whose father was a fabled Texas oilman. This nineteen-year-old received a monthly allowance of $3,500. He came to the workshop in his Turbo Porsche and when I proposed that he would have to pay a dollar a stutter, his response was, "Dr. Schwartz, that ain't no money!" To which I replied, "Roger, for you it's fifty dollars a stutter!" To which he replied, "More like it sir!"

Patients are required to practice Contract at home with someone for several months. If the exercise is done with a close friend or spouse, the money, instead of being given to that individual, is simply to be thrown out the window. The thought of doing this clearly has the potential of upsetting both parties and increases the motivation for careful attention to technique. Patients learn and practice Contract at the workshop and many have found it helpful in dealing with stressful situations long after the workshop is over.

One patient called the center to tell me about a job interview he had gone for. As the interviewer began to ask the first question, it struck my patient that the situation was like Contract and he instantly went into what he called "Contract mode." I asked him what he meant by that and he replied that it was a psychological space he was in when under Contract—a space associated with a powerfully focused attention to technique. In this space, nothing could throw him. Needless to say, insofar as speech was concerned, the interview went perfectly.

Toughening

Another exercise that has proved extremely effective is called "toughening." It is designed to make the stutterer resistant to the speed of the speech of those around him. If one is spoken to quickly, there is a tendency to respond quickly. But if a stutterer responds quickly, he will scarcely leave time for implementation of technique. Time is required to let a small bit of air flow out passively from the mouth and to slow the first word. Toughening teaches the stutterer to take this time.

Like Contract, toughening requires the presence of another person. The other person asks a question, which the patient then answers in a single sentence, employing the airflow technique. In the middle of the sentence, the assistant interrupts with a second question. The patient has to stop in mid-answer, generate another airflow, and, employing a complete sentence, respond—whereupon in mid-sentence he is again interrupted. This goes on for one minute. The patient tends to speed, discarding his technique in responding to the rapid-fire questioning. The goal is to retain the passive airflow and continue to slow the first word regardless of the speed of the question.

I frequently tell patients at workshops that, in a sense, I wish they would all develop a peculiar form of paranoia. I wish they would believe that everyone in the world was being paid by me to toughen them. This would put them on their guard and make them highly resistant to the verbal speed demands of the world around them.

11 *Basic Training*

THE AIRFLOW technique is like a sport. Small muscles are involved rather than large ones, but the same rules apply—and the first and foremost rule is to practice. The stutterer must develop a winning skill, a habit strong enough to compete successfully against the innate tendency to lock the cords. This habit must be made automatic and must look and sound natural. It takes time to achieve this—typically twelve to fifteen weeks. I call this period "basic training."

Patients are encouraged to imagine themselves as machines sitting in a room generating one perfect sentence after another, taking time between each sentence to set themselves up properly to produce the best possible example of technique. The axiom of quality rather than quantity is reinforced.

Foundation exercises
The first four weeks of basic training are devoted to foundation exercises. In these, the patient must demonstrate an absolutely consistent use of flutter and slowed first words on short, simple sentences and short speeches composed of simple sentences. This phase is critical because it constitutes the basis for subsequent progress. If there is the slightest imperfection in technique, any stress will ex-

aggerate it, and can lead to stuttering. In order to build a permanent edifice of totally fluent speech, the patient must have a completely sound foundation.

Bridging exercises
The next four or five weeks are devoted to using the technique in structured, real-life situations. These are called "bridging exercises." The goal here is to bridge the basic practice exercises into the real world. These exercises are performed with a friend, family member, or coworker.

One device that we have found helpful to patients at this stage of treatment is called the MotivAider. This is an electronic timer that looks like a personal pager and can be attached to a belt or slipped into a pocket. The MotivAider can be programmed to go off at any interval from once a minute to once a day and, when activated, produces a half-second-long vibration, reminding the patient to attend to technique.

The MotivAider was invented by Dr. Steve Levinson, a clinical psychologist in Minnesota. In a study made in 1984, he worked with a group of depressed patients who were constantly thinking depressing thoughts. He selected a positive statement and required these patients to repeat it aloud fifty times each day for several days. After that they were given the MotivAider. Each time the MotivAider went off, they were to repeat the positive statement to themselves as a thought. The chain of continuous negative thinking was thus broken at regular intervals and the depression lifted for a certain number of patients.

In our program, the MotivAider is set to go off once every three minutes and is used for three hours a day for three weeks. Each time it goes off the patient is trained to think, "The next sentence is with perfect technique." After the three-week period, the patient goes on vacation for a week and then resumes use. It has been found that several three-week cycles of MotivAider use are all that are required to make a permanent habit of the airflow technique.

During MotivAider use we introduce the concept of nickel-and-dime practice. The term "nickel-and-dime" refers to the fact that during the course of the day one can always find a spare five or ten minutes to practice. For example, many people commute to work by car. A typical trip may last twenty to forty minutes each way. During this time one is captive. What a perfect place to practice!

In the car the patient is required to generate strings of unrelated sentences. It has been estimated that if a patient drives an average of an hour a day, he can produce approximately five thousand practice sentences a week—in that one location alone!

One patient generated sentences while watching television commercials. Another practiced each time he went to the toilet. And a youngster reported nickel-and-diming during chores.

There are three types of nickel-and-dime practice. The first is called "out loud." In this, the patient uses perfect technique (a passive airflow followed by a slowed first word) to generate a series of sentences out loud.

The second type is called "silent," and in it the patient practices silently. The airflow still emerges passively, the first word is still spoken slowly, but the articulations are unaccompanied by vocal-cord vibration. Silent nickel-and-dime practice can be used in public situations where the audible production of unrelated sentences would be inappropriate or distracting to others.

The third form of nickel-and-dime practice is called "silent and covered." In it, the patient repeats silent nickel-and-dime practice but in addition covers his mouth with his hand, looks up at the ceiling, and appears to be thinking. This can be done anywhere, in virtually any situation. Of course, since the speech is silent and no one knows about it, there is no stuttering. But it doesn't matter; the patient is actually starting to get better in that situation. He is taking practice swings on his turf. And if someone comes up to him and asks him a question, it's more of the same, but out loud.

In this bridging phase of basic training the patient begins to show signs of automatic use of the technique. He reports speaking for an hour and discovering that he has been using technique without actually being conscious of precisely when he began to use it. He experiences a greater frequency of real-world successes. He begins to see that the technique *really* has the power to stop his stuttering, that it is not merely something that works in carefully structured situations, but has definite, practical applications. As all this becomes manifest, his motivation starts to soar as he begins to see the light at the end of the tunnel.

Real-world exercises
The third and final stage of basic training has been developed to confirm the stutterer's technique in any and all situations. Here are the "real-world exercises." All of the prior weeks' practice can now be seen to have been a preparation. This is the stepping-off point for the future.

We introduce the patient to a series of exercises which are graded along a hierarchy of distractibility, that is, in terms of their ability to distract the patient from attending to technique. First, we assign a simple conversation exercise that requires the patient to discuss some neutral or uninteresting topic with a friend. When the patient exhibits consistently perfect technique at this level, he progresses to conversations that are somewhat more distracting. For example, if the patient was interested in baseball, we would have him discuss the World Series. Again, the requirement for consistency of technique is strongly reinforced.

Next, we introduce the joke-telling exercise. As might be expected, stutterers report that telling jokes is difficult—

particularly when it comes to the punch line. The punch line can make or break the joke, and so it is usually a high-stress utterance, one associated with more tension on the vocal cords. In addition, amateur joke tellers tend to deliver punch lines quickly—and this raises vocal-cord tension as well.

Patients are assigned the task of telling jokes to a variety of people. Samples are recorded and sent to the center for evaluation. Occasionally one hears a burst of laughter coming from a therapy room where a therapist is monitoring tape cassettes sent by patients to the center. One can be fairly certain she is listening to jokes.

After jokes come debates. In these, the patient is required to take a position on a subject of great personal interest and to argue his position with an opponent. Often debates are held under Contract. If a patient becomes distracted and forgets to use technique, he must pay for his oversight. Debates are the most powerful of the distraction exercises, and successful mastery of them signals the completion of the last phase of basic training.

THE PATIENT now has an automatic and powerful habit. The next step is to eliminate the habit of scanning—the process of looking ahead for feared sounds, words, or speaking situations. I have found that if a patient stops practicing airflow technique when he no longer stutters but still looks ahead, he runs a substantial risk of having a relapse. All vestiges of anticipatory stress must be eliminated to ensure a permanent result.

12 *Overcoming Anticipatory Stress*

CONSISTENT USE of the airflow technique brings total fluency in a short amount of time. Patients are delighted with an easy-to-use technique that handles stuttering effortlessly. And many patients report that following the twelve- to fifteen-week period of basic training, the habit is both automatic and strong.

But it is not always that simple. Patients' use of technique is frequently compromised by the extreme stress associated with certain sounds, words, and situations. The same fears which formerly had been directly responsible for the locking of the vocal cords now produce the same locking indirectly—by completely filling the patient's conscious awareness and preventing attention to the technique. The result is inevitable: the patient stutters, which, in turn, raises stress further, leading to still more difficulty. Early success is reversed by a tenacious array of anticipatory stresses.

In order to secure fluency, patients need to be able to handle these stresses consistently. Indeed, it is the elimination of these speaking fears and scanning behaviors, rather than the initial fluency produced by mastering the airflow technique, that signals the permanent result.

These fears will not abate by themselves, however, and merely wishing them away won't work. They need conscious attention—a deliberate, planned strategy—and sometimes they take months to overcome. Of course, everyone has his own personal methods for dealing with stress, but here are two we have found to be particularly effective in dealing with anticipatory stress in stutterers.

Systematic desensitization
Developed by psychologists to help patients overcome specific situation fears, systematic desensitization involves creating a hierarchy of examples of a stress situation (from low to high), and then slowly and successfully negotiating the patient through each step to gradually build confidence. For example, if a patient reports a fear of job interviews, she will be advised to interview first for jobs that hold no interest for her. The rationale is that there will be virtually no stress associated with the interview. After handling these interviews successfully, the patient will be encouraged to interview for positions that she finds more attractive. The hierarchy is obvious: the least desirable position will be interviewed for first, the most desirable one will be reserved for last. And after a week or two, if the hierarchical steps are chosen properly, the fear of job-interviewing should be extinguished.

I have found this procedure to be very effective in eliminating anticipatory stress in stutterers. An example shows the process in detail. Several years ago I treated a man from New Jersey who, in spite of a severe stutter, had managed to develop a successful automobile dealership. Now, at forty, he seriously wished to marry and have a family. But he always stuttered severely when meeting women socially.

He suffered from an interesting if not altogether unusual hierarchical affliction: the prettier the woman, the greater the stress and the more he stuttered.

He confided this dilemma to me one morning as we sat in my office. The description of his fear hierarchy prompted an idea. I suggested that we visit a series of bars. I would choose the bars and he would engage in a systematic desensitization while we bar-hopped. He agreed to the proposal.

At the appointed time and location, in a somewhat disreputable part of town, we entered a bar, and I pointed to a "bag lady" sitting disconsolately in a corner. My patient, when told to approach her with an offer of a drink, balked, saying that this was not a stressful situation since the woman was unattractive. My response was that this was a fine place to begin.

He approached the woman, bought a drink and offered it to her. The conversation was brief and the technique excellent. No stuttering occurred.

At our next location we encountered a fiftyish woman of obvious means but with a clear addiction to alcohol. She had already had several drinks and was intoxicated as my patient sidled up to her to engage in conversation. Again the technique was employed and again fluent speech ensued. Later I pointed out that this woman was far more attractive than the one he had spoken with just twenty minutes earlier and that, as a result, we should proceed to the next step.

A taxi ride to the other side of town brought us to a favorite after-work spot frequented by secretaries and young executives who worked in the many office buildings in the neighborhood. We chose as our next "victim" a woman in her late thirties who, while sober and moderately attractive, was not too eager to speak with my patient since she was looking for a friend. He persisted, however, and found that he could still attend to technique in spite of the fact that she showed no real interest in him. He reported later that he had been on edge but had managed to hold on to technique.

I decided not to proceed further up the hierarchy at this point, and chose another woman about the same age who seemed both single and more self-contained. My patient found in her an immediate conversation partner and spoke at length. After the conversation he reported that his stress was again low. I noted to him that this woman was very attractive and he acknowledged this with a smile.

In the next bar he soloed. As soon as we had selected our person, I left and it was his task to both initiate conversation and sustain it with perfect technique. I chose a remarkably attractive woman and left. Twenty minutes later my patient skipped out of the bar in obvious delight and as he approached, pulled a slip of paper from his pocket—the woman had given him her phone number!

The night was young and I suggested that he continue to practice in as many bars as he could find until his fear was completely gone. This he agreed to do, and in the course of the next several days he extinguished a lifelong fear. Two and a half years later I attended his wedding.

The same hierarchical procedure can be applied to deal with word or sound fears. A common example is the difficulty some stutterers have saying their name. The reason is obvious: one cannot word-substitute one's name and it is often the first thing said in a conversation, where the peak of the stress is greatest. Many stutterers remember sitting in a classroom on the first day of school as the teacher went around the room having the students say their names. As their turn approached, the stress mounted to horrific proportions and the result was always a stutter.

With such a history it is no wonder that some patients, in order to avoid stuttering on their name, either always spell it or never leave home without a business card. One patient went so far as to have his name changed to one which he could say easily, only to discover that the stress had now shifted and he could not say his new name.

The solution to this problem of saying a feared word

such as one's name is first to practice saying it *with perfect technique a thousand times.* Employing a leisurely pace and practicing approximately a half hour a day for four days will produce the required number of repetitions. Following this, the patient is encouraged to repeat his name with perfect technique to the closest person he knows, whether a spouse, parent, or best friend. Twenty-five repetitions per day for a week will suffice. The patient is to increase every day the number of people with whom this practice is performed.

The hierarchical concept is at work here since the patient starts first with the easiest, least fearsome person and then progresses to more and more difficult ones.

The next step is to use lists of 800 numbers to make calls. When the operator responds, the patient is required, with perfect technique, to say his name and hang up. This may appear rude, but I have always justified the operator's momentary minor inconvenience by the benefit to the patient's life.

The next step is to begin mentioning one's name in conversation. For example, a patient will talk about a hard-of-hearing grandparent who could not comprehend speech over the telephone. In the course of telling the story he will say: "I kept on telling him, 'Grandpa, this is me, John Smith.' " Whether or not John Smith really has a hard-of-hearing grandfather is immaterial; the fact is that he is saying his name in conversation.

I've had patients page themselves at airports, call information for their phone numbers, and call hotels to find out if someone with their name is registered. One patient even made up a fictitious company name which was in fact his own, and used this to describe a wonderful stock investment he had heard about. Of course, this ruse worked only with strangers!

There seems to be great variability in the number of successful experiences people need to become convinced that they no longer have to look ahead for feared words or sounds. Some individuals are highly suggestible—a few instances are all it takes to persuade them. Others have anticipatory stresses that linger for weeks or months before finally being extinguished.

The Callahan technique

About ten years ago, Dr. Roger Callahan, a clinical psychologist in southern California, made a rather remarkable discovery. Using a technique developed originally by exercise physiologists, he was able to identify certain places on the body, known as *meridians*, that were associated with fear reactions. By using a modified form of acupressure which involves percussively tapping on these meridians with the fingertips, he found that he could treat phobic reactions that had existed for years in as little as ten minutes, and that these reactions often did not return.

After reading his book, *The Five Minute Phobia Cure*, I thought about applying his methods to my work with stutterers. Here, it seemed, was a way of treating speaking fears that could possibly be used as a complement, even an alternative, to the systematic desensitization procedure. I arranged to sit in on one of his treatment sessions, and was able to see a number of demonstrations of the power of his technique.

For example, knowing that one of the patients scheduled to be seen that day had a morbid fear of spiders, he had gone to his garden, captured one, and placed it in a cardboard box. He concealed the box in his desk drawer when the woman arrived. After a brief interview, he produced the spider and the woman exhibited a strong panic reaction.

Replacing the box and its contents in his drawer, he spent the next six minutes showing her the technique, teaching her how and where to tap her acupressure meridians. Then he removed the box and dumped the spider into her palm. I head her mutter, "I can't believe I'm doing this! I can't believe I'm doing this!" The spider slowly walked on her hand until she calmly restored it to its cardboard enclosure.

I questioned her about her fear. Had she always been afraid of spiders? Could she explain her apparent tranquillity? She had no answers for me. And more important, she acted as if this total extinction of fear was a natural occurrence, something to be expected.

When she left, I asked Callahan about her apparently blasé reaction to what must have been a monumental accomplishment for her—the elimination of a major lifelong fear. He told me that his patients generally were unwilling to acknowledge that such a dramatic change could be brought about simply by tapping a few selected areas on the surface of the body.

The next patient reported a profound fear of heights. She had avoided stairs for years, and sometimes this created serious problems. For example, she had attended a movie the week before and was unable to go to the toilet because it required walking up stairs.

Callahan produced a stepladder and asked her to climb the first step. She appeared emotionally shaken but complied with his request. At the suggestion that she mount the next step, she not only refused but stepped back to the ground.

Callahan immediately went to work, and after five minutes she climbed straight to the top of the ladder and showed not a trace of her former fear.

Was this a setup? Was I being duped? How could a lifelong fear be treated in five minutes? And for eighty percent of these people, Callahan assured me, the treatment would be permanent, with the remaining twenty percent requiring several sessions.

Callahan's explanation of the results in terms of blocked energy flows in the body left much to be desired. It seemed to me that there was no scientific basis for his conclusions; it was all pure conjecture. On the other hand, his apparent successes could not be ignored.

Was the fear of speaking in certain situations reported by stutterers amenable to the Callahan technique? I posed the question to him and he responded that a fear is a fear and that all fears could be directly dealt with using his method.

The day after I observed the treatment session, Callahan taught me how to teach the technique. Though I discovered that each patient requires a somewhat different approach, in all cases the technique can be taught in less than fifteen minutes.

One day I received a phone call from a thirty-seven-year-old woman who had been a patient of mine for approximately two months. The occupation she had chosen, working in a typing pool for a major corporation, required minimal verbal interaction. She had started out a severe stutterer, had mastered the basic foundation exercises, and was on her way to bridging them into the real world. During this time she had secured a position as secretary and now, at 9:30 on a Monday morning, she was panicked by the requirement of answering the incessant stream of phone calls coming in to her employer. We had not yet practiced phone work and she had stuttered a great deal on the phone during the first ten minutes on the job. She knew that if this continued she would be fired.

I suggested that she "get sick," leave the office, and come immediately to my office. When she arrived, I began the Callahan technique. I showed her a couple of acupressure points, one under the eyes and another on top of the hand. She tapped these vigorously and her fears seemed to abate. We tried the phone and found that she was able to use the airflow technique to speak with a seeming sense of utter tranquillity.

I suggested she practice both the Callahan and airflow

techniques on the telephone at home for the rest of the day. I gave her a lengthy list of 800 numbers to use. I further suggested that she practice the Callahan procedure the following morning in the ladies' room before starting work. I told her to call me mid-morning.

At 4:30 P.M. the next day I still had not heard from her. I called her office and she answered the phone perfectly. When I asked her about her fear level, she replied, "Oh that—it's completely gone."

This woman's story is representative of the dramatic successes that many stutterers have had with the Callahan technique. But a word of caution: although Callahan says he has used his technique for over a decade, it is still relatively new in the treatment of stuttering. The technique appears extremely promising, and is being considered as an alternative to the longer-duration systematic desensitization procedures. But until we are able to do follow-up studies to ensure the permanence of the result, I continue to use both Callahan's approach and the slower systematic desensitization technique with all patients.

13 *Preventing Relapse*

IRONICALLY, ONE of the greatest advantages of the passive airflow technique—the speed with which it often brings total fluency—can, with some patients, also be one of its greatest drawbacks. A patient who on Monday had been a severe stutterer may, on Tuesday, speak effortlessly everywhere without a trace of his former problem. He, his friends, and family would be delighted; his therapist, on the other hand, would be deeply concerned.

For the immediate success produced by the airflow technique in some patients can be reversed as quickly as it was learned, if careful maintenance is ignored. A highly suggestible patient, having just overcome a major life-long difficulty, may let down his defenses and relax his attention to technique, and in doing so run the risk of having his stuttering return at the slightest provocation. He also opens himself up to another, more subtle, complication—a condition that I call "the assault of the subconscious."

The assault of the subconscious occurs only in individuals with a moderate or severe stutter who quickly become fluent. Shortly after attaining fluency the patient reports experiencing an anxiety attack which may range from nervousness to a deeper sense of dread. The anxiety continues unabated for days and the patient begins to feel that if only he were to start stuttering again, his anxieties would subside. For a small percentage of patients the stress is so great they succumb to the temptation. The stress does indeed stop after the resumption of stuttering and the patient vows "never to go near that fluency again."

The theoretical explanation for the assault of the subconscious is as follows: The subconscious plays a critical role in producing and maintaining a person's identity. In a person who stutters, the subconscious sees itself as a stutterer. For years the individual has been telling his subconscious that he cannot say certain sounds, certain words, or speak in certain situations—and the subconscious believes it. The subconscious does not place a value judgment on stuttering, it simply says that's the way it is. Value judgments come from the conscious mind.

When a person abruptly stops stuttering, the subconscious becomes disoriented. Fluency is not the normal state of affairs. The subconscious becomes "concerned" that the well-being of the individual is being threatened, and it tries to restore its self-concept as a stutterer by raising the person's level of anxiety.

It is well known in learning psychology that all newly acquired behaviors are easily lost under conditions of stress. The passive airflow technique is no exception. The elevated state of anxiety is an attempt on the part of the subconscious to convince the individual to give up his newly learned fluency.

During my early experiences with stutterers I found that fully a third of those who became totally fluent quickly reported the assault of the subconscious. Some would hang tough and after a week or two the anxiety attacks would be gone; others would succumb to the temptation to resume stuttering and soon would be lost to the program. I have come to recognize the assault of the subconscious as the precipitating cause of relapse in patients who attain total fluency quickly.

The bathtub technique

The "bathtub technique" is a treatment that has been developed by the National Center for Stuttering to deal with the assault of the subconscious. At first it may seem unusual, but it has been used with over four thousand patients and it works.

Three things are required: a bathtub filled with warm water, a candle in a candle holder, and a mirror. The candle is lit, placed in the holder, and put on the ledge of the tub. The mirror is placed next to it. The patient then turns out the light, enters the tub, lies back in the water so that his torso is completely submerged, breathes calmly in and out through his nose, and stares at a spot on the wall directly in front of him. Each time the air comes out of his nose, he thinks the word "one." As he does this, he may find his mind starting to drift, starting to think other thoughts. Each time this happens, he is to bring his mind gently back to thinking the word "one." Since the mind is an undisciplined thing, he may find himself frequently having to bring it back to the thought. But he is to persevere for at least five minutes and steep there in the tub like a pot of tea.

Here's how the first phase of this technique works: First, the warm water mechanically relaxes the muscles of the body. Second, the subdued light from the candle prevents any bright light from tensing the patient's eyes. Third, fixing his eyes on a spot on the wall prevents scanning movements, which is important to this exercise since scanning movements have been shown to stimulate muscle tension. Fourth, thinking the word "one" over and over again renders the word meaningless, like repeating a Hindu mantra, and this prevents the patient from thinking about what he should have done yesterday and what he has to do tomorrow. Such thoughts stimulate tension too.

In those five minutes, we are attempting to strip away

as much muscle tension as we can, to create as much of an intrauterine experience as we can, our mother's uterus being the safest place we've ever known—warm, moist, dark, supportive, thoughtless, relaxed. We are using an intrauterine model as the physiological rationale for this first phase of the bathtub technique.

We now move to the second phase. The patient sits up in the tub, picks up the mirror, and positions it so that he can see his eyes. Using perfect airflow technique, he begins to repeat the word "relax" slowly, using an extremely soft voice. He does this for about three minutes (usually about fifty repetitions are produced during this time). These first two phases are designed to reduce muscle tension to a level where we can access the subconscious.

We are now ready for the third and most important phase of the program. In it, the patient is literally going to brainwash himself: he is going to change the self-concept of the subconscious.

The patient reads a specially prepared series of positive statements called *affirmations.* The affirmations are prepared individually for each patient. For example, for one particularly high-stress patient the affirmations may focus on relaxation: *"As I practice I become more and more relaxed."* For another, the emphasis may be on building self-esteem: *"My confidence is growing higher and higher each day."* These affirmations are read three times using the airflow technique. One affirmation is designed to provide subconscious motivation to practice. It is naïve to rely solely on conscious desire when the subconscious is free and accessible.

Each patient is also provided with a cue word to say silently before entering a stressful speaking situation. Many stutterers, when they say the cue word, experience a profound drop in overall tension—to the point where they feel as if they are alone, even if they are in the middle of a large group. Their fluency is then assured.

14 *Support Systems*

Stutterers rarely, if ever, stutter when they talk to themselves out loud alone. Therefore, any attempt to make a permanent change must consider the outside world—that is, the world of speaking individuals. It is terribly difficult for someone who has stuttered his whole life to suddenly communicate fluently with others, and sometimes the strain is so great that the patient suffers a relapse and begins stuttering all over again. Knowledgeable friends and family members can offer reassurance and reinforcement, but we have discovered that a more systematic program is what is most effective. Indeed, to assure permanent fluency in any and all situations, a treatment program should continue to offer follow-up long after the stutterer has demonstrated fluency in the classroom and at home or work.

Among the many follow-up resources available is the system of reinforcements developed by the National Center for Stuttering over the past fifteen years to assist stutterers in transition and help them maintain fluency. This program is offered through a nationwide network, enabling patients living anywhere in the United States to refresh their technique and get moral support from professionals and other stutterers. Patients have found this support network extremely helpful, and it has become an integral part of the NCS program.

Therapists
Ongoing support from a speech therapist can be invaluable. Our patients participate in an active exchange process with a trained therapist for nine to twelve months after basic training is over. The therapist monitors the patient's performance weekly via a cassette tape, and guides him through difficult speaking situations.

While one can learn to stop stuttering completely in a few short months, anticipatory stress—the habit of scanning ahead for feared sounds, words, or speaking situations—can take longer to overcome. The patient's "scanner" must be put to sleep, and since it is deeply imbedded in his subconscious this can be a complex psychological process. The stutterer must be patient. In the course of working with thousands of stutterers, I have learned that if a patient stops practicing the airflow technique when he no longer stutters, but still scans, his risk of having a relapse is great. Having the ongoing support of a therapist gives many patients the extra incentive they need to stick with the program.

Refresher courses
Many stutterers have found refresher courses invaluable for brushing up on technique and renewing motivation to practice. The National Center for Stuttering offers refresher courses periodically throughout the United States, giving patients face-to-face contact with a therapist. These courses allow time for dealing in depth with particular questions raised by patients, and provide an opportunity to discuss highly refined strategies for handling unusual and high-stress speaking situations.

For example, one patient worked in a nuclear electric generating plant. He was an evening supervisor and virtually ran the plant. His stuttering was controlled, but his greatest fear was that in the event of a crisis, when called upon to give a long and complex series of commands rapidly, he would be unable to do so. He lived in fear that if a crisis did occur, it would prove devastating not only to him but to those who relied on him. This knowledge weighed heavily upon him, and he thought a great deal about changing jobs.

He came to a refresher course and I suggested that he stage simulated emergencies or full-blown dress rehearsals on a regular basis. Emergency drills were, of course, routine procedure at the nuclear installation, but by increasing their frequency and making them as vivid as possible, he would be able to practice speaking under pressure, and learn to control the emotional responses that might occur in such a situation.

Six months later I received a letter from him telling me that there had been a true emergency at the plant, and that he had handled it flawlessly. Not only had he achieved a personal victory, but he had also been promoted to a new position—one that did not require him to speak under stress.

The National Stutterers' Hotline: 1-800-221-2483
One component of our support network that has helped countless stutterers with their problems is the special hotline number. This toll-free service is staffed by trained professionals, and is available to anyone who stutters, or his family or friends. It is extremely comforting to know that a knowledgeable therapist is available to provide support and advice. *If you stutter or know someone who does, you are encouraged to call the hotline for information concerning the availability of treatment programs in your area.*

In the past, stutterers have called about particular assignments, or if they are having a bad day, or if they are worried about an upcoming speaking situation and want a strategy for maximizing their success, or if they are in an emergency situation and need help—quick! For example, several years ago I treated a patient who worked for the State Department. He had performed reasonably well in his career because he was a closet stutterer. But he was hampered by his inability to learn a second language, which is a requirement for advancement in the State Department. The difficulty was that in the second language he did not have the facility to word-substitute. He would have to say all of the feared sounds, and his anxiety over this prospect had grown to gargantuan proportions; the mere thought of having to study a foreign language was terrifying.

In the State Department intensive foreign language courses are provided in which one can study six hours a day for a number of weeks until mastery of the basic elements of conversation is achieved. My patient wanted to learn French, but all his past attempts had failed miserably. Now he had been practicing the airflow technique for six months and felt he was ready.

The first day of training began. The session went well for the first half hour, and then he hit his first serious block on a *t* sound. He suddenly became extremely anxious and found himself unable to continue. All his old fears about learning a second language returned with full force.

He asked to be excused, went to the nearest pay phone, and dialed the toll-free hotline number. A therapist responded and counseled him about both technique and strategy. She reviewed the basic features of the technique and suggested he return to class, but speak softly and slowly for the rest of the day. She also suggested that he inform his instructor that he would be speaking in this manner. He was told to call back as often as necessary. On the first day he called a number of times; on the second, twice. He successfully completed the course.

While technical support of the type provided by our therapists, refresher courses, and the National Stutterers' Hotline has proven extremely effective in helping former stutterers remain fluent we've found that it is other stutterers' successes that provide the real psychological edge, the greatest hope and motivation to stutterers still working to overcome their affliction. Let's consider some of the other support programs that have proven effective.

Clubs
Sharing a problem with others who are working through a similar situation can be invaluable. Clubs for airflow users have been established in most major cities in the United States. These generally meet twice a month in local hospitals, churches, or libraries and serve as powerful support groups. A rotating leadership system allows each member to lead meetings, and members perform various exercises to refresh their technique. Most importantly, they are able to share their stories of victory and defeat with people who really understand. This mutual support provides members with maximum motivation to continue practicing the airflow technique on a daily basis.

Advanced club members often function as a sort of miniature lecture bureau. They arrange to give group lectures on stuttering to various local organizations, such as speech-therapy classes at local colleges or women's groups. Their goal is not only to educate a public that needs such knowledge, but in the process to use the support of the club as a tool to broaden their own public-speaking experience and gain self-confidence. Newer members in the club aspire to join these mini-lecture bureaus and, once they have become sufficiently expert in the use of the technique, are welcomed into the bureau.

Many club members have also given interviews to local newspapers and have spoken on radio and television. The change in self-concept from being a person who stutters to a person who receives applause for a public lecture is one of the most dramatic possible. An individual who accomplishes this goal has gone so far psychologically that the possibility of relapse is extremely remote.

Many of the participants in these club meetings go on to

join a national public-speaking organization called Toast-masters. There they have an opportunity to give a speech before an audience every week. A number of airflowers have become presidents of their local Toastmasters chapters, and others have won regional public-speaking competitions.

The monitor system

Another helpful technique draws on the age-old concept of the buddy system. We call it the monitor system—a monitor being a person (spouse, parent, or friend) who has a vital interest in the stutterer.

A monitor totally understands the stutterer's treatment program. He may practice the airflow technique with the patient or encourage him to confront speaking fears. He is almost like a surrogate parent, a mother or father who is intimately involved with the child's homework. We have discovered that patients make much greater progress if there is someone at home and/or work or school who is intimately involved with the rehabilitation program. People have much more power to change when they are with another person rather than alone.

From time to time a stutterer reports that he lives alone, that he knows virtually no one, that his work is done in isolation, and that he cannot think of anyone who might be a suitable monitor. I suggest that he go out and hire one, that he pay a high school student a few dollars an hour to function as a monitor. At all costs, he must not try to go it alone. He is to think of the stutterer inside himself as a sort of child—a child who needs parenting.

We have repeatedly discovered that monitors are crucial to the establishment of success and that patients who try to go it alone court disaster. Although it is possible for some individuals to succeed on their own, their number is small. The general suggestion is: get a monitor. And if you can find two, you are twice blessed.

Banquets

One of greatest satisfactions for an ex-stutterer who has triumphed over his affliction is the opportunity to share his achievement with others. Each year, throughout the United States, banquets are held in a number of cities to celebrate the achievements of airflow students. After dinner, thirty individuals present short speeches on a topic related to the theme "How My Life Has Changed." Their speeches are testimony to how far these individuals have come in changing their lives. You'll read some of these wonderful first-person success stories in Part Three of this book.

A call for speakers for an upcoming banquet is usually announced a month in advance; the first thirty to respond are chosen. In recent years, far more have responded than time allotted. Those who are "shut out" are given top priority for the following year's presentation. I recall one patient who felt so disappointed at not being able to speak at a Washington, D.C., banquet that he submitted his name for one in New York, was accepted, and flew up for the dinner.

Individuals who have shown an interest in learning airflow but have not yet done so are invited to attend a banquet and listen to the after-dinner speakers. Many of these stutterers are skeptical about being able to recover. They have tried many therapies, none of which has ever worked for any considerable amount of time. As these individuals hear one success story after another, a glimmer of hope begins to develop.

WE HAVE found these support systems absolutely critical in making success stick. Without them, patients must fend for themselves and, unfortunately, very few have enough personal resources to make such a major permanent change.

15 For Parents: Will Your Child Outgrow the Problem?

ONE OF the most important functions of the National Center for Stuttering is to counsel parents whose children have just recently begun to stutter. The onset of stuttering usually occurs between the ages of two and six, and in 70 percent of cases is spontaneously outgrown by age ten. The remaining 30 percent statistically constitute the 2.6 million Americans who stutter today.

Kids who stutter, whether or not they outgrow it spontaneously, are usually teased mercilessly by peers. It is not uncommon for them to withdraw socially and establish patterns of extremely low self-esteem. This early behavior is carried through in school and helps form the pattern of the underachiever. Many adult stutterers say that the cruel teasing from schoolmates they received as youngsters was the most painful experience associated with their affliction. It is only natural, then, for parents to try to protect their children from such misery.

Often, the first step taken by a concerned parent is to call the child's pediatrician. And invariably the pediatrician says, "Do nothing, the child will outgrow it." In most cases, this is what happens. But then there are the 30 percent who continue to stutter. What about them? And what about the years of struggle that sometimes pass before the other children eventually outgrow their stuttering?

Over the years, I have counseled thousands of parents and have developed what I call the *probability outgrowth factor.* We now are in a position to tell parents which children will spontaneously outgrow their stuttering and which may face a lifetime of stuttering if not treated by early therapy.

The probability outgrowth factor is a statistical concept. It can predict the *probability* of a child's outgrowing stuttering, but not the absolute *certainty*. Factors beyond our control—usually in the form of physical and/or emotional traumas—can blur these probabilities. Examples include serious unexpected illnesses, physical accidents such as automobile collisions, and purely emotional stresses such as parental divorce.

The probability outgrowth factor is calculated from responses to a series of questions. Each question is weighted differently in terms of importance.

1. Is there someone in the immediate family who stutters?
2. Is it a boy or a girl?
3. How old was the child when he or she began to stutter?
4. Has the stuttering been continuous or has there been a period(s) of remission?
5. Does the child have good days and bad days?
6. Does the stutter appear only at the beginning of sentences or can it appear anywhere within a sentence?
7. Is the stuttering an effortless repetition of words or sounds, or is it a strong struggle?

8. Does the child not stutter but just seem to get stuck?
9. Has the struggle been becoming more forceful?
10. Does the child appear to be conscious of his or her stuttering?
11. Does the child appear to be changing words, that is, does he sense that a difficult word is approaching and attempt to provide a synonym for it?
12. Does the child seem to be avoiding certain speaking situations?
13. Is the child using starter words or sounds like "well" or "um" in his speech?
14. Does the child appear to be unusually silent?

A parent can obtain the answers to these questions either by direct observation or by questioning the child. The parent is encouraged to call the center with these answers in hand. The results are then entered into a computer which performs a numerical analysis, yielding the probability outgrowth score.

Our analyses show that the current age of the child is a critical factor in assessing probability. For example, a seven-year-old with a 50 percent probability of outgrowth is in immediate need of attention, while a two-year-old with the same probability is merely to be monitored. Often we will tell a parent to monitor the fourteen factors at six-month intervals and submit their findings to us for recomputation. As the child gets older, the probability outgrowth factor should increase. When it does not, but instead stays level or drops, we begin to become concerned and appropriate advice is given.

Once the probability outgrowth factor has been computed, one of three courses of action is suggested. The first is to do nothing and monitor again in six months. The second is for the parents to engage in a set of activities designed to increase the probability of outgrowth (see below). And the third is to seek competent professional help.

If your child's stuttering continues to be a concern but does not yet seem serious enough to require professional help, here are seven suggestions that should help.

1. Eliminate all sources of refined sugar from the child's diet to as great an extent as possible. Young children are particularly sensitive to the tension effects of refined sugar. We recognize that it is often extremely difficult to comply with this request, but we have seen the scrupulous elimination of refined sugar either reduce or totally eliminate stuttering in a substantial number of children.

2. For the same reason, eliminate as much as possible all sources of caffeine in the diet of the young child. Caffeine is frequently present in Cola drinks and chocolate, both of which should be eliminated from the diet. Do not allow your child to drink coffee.

3. Supplement the child's diet with a good multivitamin and mineral made especially for children. Some vitamins and minerals have been shown to have a positive effect on reducing muscle tensions (including the muscles in the vocal cords) with young children. Ask your pediatrician to recommend a brand. Also, with the pediatrician's approval, add twenty milligrams of vitamin B_1 each morning. It may not be possible to obtain vitamin B_1 in dosages this small, so break the pills. For children who are unable to swallow pills or pill fragments, the vitamin may be crushed and mixed with applesauce.

4. It will be extremely helpful if both parents speak softly and slowly to the child and to others when in the child's presence. Use a confidential tone of voice, paying particular attention to the slowing of the first word of each sentence. Young children have a strong tendency to respond in kind, and if you speak softly and slowly to them, they will tend to use a similar mode of speech, and this will reduce or eliminate their stuttering.

5. Allow the child plenty of time to speak so that he does not feel he has to rush to get a word in edge-

wise. Young stuttering children often suffer from what I call verbal impetuosity, in that they feel they must rush because if they don't others will trample their words. This is seen frequently in households with a number of children all vying to be heard to get their parents' attention. It is also encountered among children of highly verbal professionals who prize large vocabularies and speedy responses.

6. **Reduce, to as great an extent as possible, all obvious sources of stress in the home and school environments.** At home this means trying to maintain an attitude of gentle caring and reducing attempts to control behavior—to give the child the sense of being heard, to be a noncritical listener, and to have the child know that you are always there for her. At school this means asking the teacher to temporarily excuse the child from having to perform orally in class. Questions may be written and submitted to the teacher, or they may be asked after class. If the teacher is cooperative, and the child would like to read aloud in class, then choral reading can be used since stutterers have no difficulty when they read aloud with others.

Most of all, it is vitally important that parents appreciate that what might appear to be a mild stutter at home can often be quite severe at school. School and home are the two most important speaking situations for children, and concern for one at the expense of the other ultimately helps perpetuate the stuttering.

7. **If the child appears to be unaware of his speech problem, do not call it to his attention.** However, if he appears to be aware of it and comes to you for help, suggest that he speak softly and slowly, particularly slowing the first word of each sentence. Using a confidential tone of voice, demonstrate this mode of speech to him. Call it "the good speech" and suggest that if he uses the good speech, most of his difficulty can be eliminated. If the child can read, it helps to mark the first word of each sentence

to indicate that it is to be read slowly and to write the word "softly" in red ink at the top of each page to remind him to speak more softly in general. Have your child read to you from his "good speech" book for five or ten minutes each day, sitting in a special chair he's chosen to be the "good speech chair." The reading and the chair will then become generally associated with fluent speech. Gradually enlarge the "good speech environment" from the "good speech chair" to the "good speech room" to the "good speech apartment" (or house) and finally to the "good speech world." Remember, it is very difficult for a young child to use the "good speech" when all around him people are speaking loudly and rapidly. As parents, you are the most important speech models and must not lose sight of this responsibility.

These and other suggestions are provided to parents by the National Center for Stuttering when they call the special hotline number (1-800-221-2483). It must be pointed out, however, that these suggestions will not work if the child displays severe struggles and/or the ability to anticipate the feared words and sounds approaching. The probability outgrowth factor for such children will usually be poor since the tension on the vocal cords is so great that speaking softly and slowing the first word will be insufficient to keep them from locking. In such cases, the airflow technique will be required.

Children as young as five can make use of the airflow technique provided they are taught by a competent therapist and one or both of the parents is actively engaged on a daily basis in the therapeutic process. If a therapist trained in these methods cannot be found, then try to find a local speech therapist and ask her or him to contact the center with a view toward participating in one of our regional therapist-training seminars. Then, as part of the training, the therapist can work with your child and his progress can also be monitored by the center.

Children older than seven can participate directly in one of the regional treatment workshops provided by the center throughout the year. With one or both parents present, the family will learn the techniques for stopping stuttering and reducing stress, and through a tape monitoring procedure will be counseled and guided through the procedures required to produce permanent fluency.

16 *Selecting a Treatment Program*

BECAUSE OF the time required to train a therapist, it is not surprising that a number of centers professing to use an airflow technique do not. Here are some guidelines to use when selecting a program.

1. Ask whether a member of the staff has been certified by the National Center for Stuttering as an airflow therapist. Frequently therapists profess to use an airflow technique after simply hearing it described by a colleague.

2. Ask to speak to patients who have been through the program to determine what their results have been. Be especially interested in long-term results. Ask to speak with a patient treated at least two years earlier.

3. Inquire as to what kind of long-term follow-up support system is provided. Patients are fragile and can easily recondition their old fears and relapse. They must be monitored for months.

4. Be skeptical of any program that promises to achieve permanent changes in a few weeks; it is absolutely unrealistic to expect that a lifelong problem will be changed so quickly.

5. Ask whether the program considers the importance of base-level stress and its variability as an integral component of their treatment approach. If not, then a major contributor to the tension on the vocal cords is being neglected.
6. If any doubt exists about the competence of the program, call the National Center for Stuttering for an opinion.

There are so many different clinicians employing such a variety of approaches that it is often difficult to evaluate them all properly. But some definite conclusions can be drawn. Any program, if it is good, will produce an initial fluency quickly. If the technique does not accomplish this, the program should be discontinued. Similarly, stutterers should avoid a clinician who does not specialize in stuttering but instead treats a variety of speech or psychological problems. Stuttering is a specialized area, and its treatment is best left to those with extensive clinical experience. Finally, no therapy should be pursued if the clinician cannot offer a numerical probability of likely eventual success.

17 *Ongoing Research for Treatment*

W**HAT DOES** the future hold? Much promise, I think. The creation of the National Institute of Deafness and Communication Disorders in Washington, D.C. has ensured substantial and continued federal funding for research into stuttering.

We are beginning to see the results of this research. In 1989 several investigators reported discovering the area in the brain responsible for the locking of the vocal cords in stutterers. This finding means that researchers may now begin to attempt to develop medications targeted to work in that area. It is conceivable that in the future, stuttering might be treated by the simple expedient of taking a pill.

Researchers at the National Institutes of Health are attempting to deal with the problem of stuttering by injecting a chemical substance into the muscles which move the vocal cords. This substance acts to temporarily weaken or paralyze the cords, thus preventing them from locking. Preliminary findings have shown some reduction of stuttering and further research is under way with larger numbers of patients. It seems likely that one future approach to the treatment of stuttering may involve injections to the vocal cords once or twice a year. Most individuals who stutter would probably be willing to undergo this procedure if they knew it to be effective.

Perhaps the most exciting line of research currently under way is based on a study recently conducted by the National Center for Stuttering in conjunction with a major New York hospital. In this study, we anesthetized the vocal cords in a group of four stutterers to determine if we could eliminate the neurological trigger for stuttering—the nerve impulses that report vocal-cord tension to the brain. If the brain never realized there was tension on the vocal cords, stuttering could be avoided.

The nerves in the vocal cords are intricate mechanisms that actually serve two functions. On the one hand, they are sensory nerves, detecting tension within the vocal-cord muscles and sending this information to the brain. On the other hand, they are also motor nerves, receiving impulses from the brain which instruct the vocal cords to contract or relax. Any procedure designed to numb the nerves must be able to isolate the sensory portion of the nerve, for numbing the motor portion as well would result in paralysis of the cords and then, of course, speech would be impossible.

Fortunately, the fibers within the nerve are arranged in such a way that we can selectively target the sensory function. The motor fibers carrying nerve impulses *to* the muscles are clustered together in the center, while the sensory fibers carrying nerve impulses *from* the muscles are arranged on the outer surface. When a nerve is injected with anesthetic, it is initially blocked in both directions, but after a period of time, usually about twenty minutes, the inner core (motor portion) recovers, followed by the outer surface. If our thinking was correct, injection to the nerves on both sides would result in immediate total paralysis of the cords, followed by initial return of the motor ability to tense the cords and then a return of sensation from the cords.

In all, four adult stutterers received the injections. The first, a man of about forty-five, suffered from a severe stutter of lifelong duration. Ten minutes after receiving the bilateral injections he became aphonic—that is, he was unable to make any sound whatsoever; his paralyzed cords were too weak to approximate one another. He was able to mouth his words, but they were rendered in silence.

Thirty-seven minutes following the injection a weak, breathy voice started to be heard. Over the next twenty-six minutes the voice became progressively stronger as the anesthetic in the inner core of both nerves wore off.

The remarkable aspect of this patient's speech was that during the twenty-six-minute period he was totally fluent—not only on words spoken in isolation, but also in sentences, ongoing conversations, and even telephone calls. After this period of fluency, he gradually began to stutter as the sensory portion of his nerve recovered from the effects of the anesthetic. During the next twelve minutes he completely relapsed into his former stuttering pattern.

The other three patients in the study demonstrated similar responses: first total loss of voice, followed by a weak but fluent voice which regained strength progressively, and finally an initial mild stutter which over a relatively short period of time attained its pre-anesthetic level of severity.

This finding confirmed our hypothesis that if we could selectively block the outer, sensory, surface of the nerve fibers going to the vocal cords, we could probably eliminate stuttering.

One of my colleagues at New York University is now working on just such an approach. The work is still at the test-tube stage. Small portions of mixed nerves taken from animals are being kept alive in supportive media while a variety of enzymes are being applied to the nerves. Some of these enzymes have an affinity for sensory nerves—in a sense, they eat them. Studies are under way to find the best approach that most cleanly eliminates the sensory nerves while leaving the motor portions intact.

The implication of this line of inquiry is obvious: if we can prevent the brain from receiving sensory information from the vocal cords, we will have removed the trigger for stuttering and there will be no stuttering. Furthermore, all that would likely be required would be a single injection on either side of the larynx, administered once. The patient would be rendered fluent on a permanent basis.

In another area of research, it has been shown that if a stutterer speaks against a very loud background noise, the stuttering tends to be totally eliminated. Indeed, in the ancient literature on stuttering there is occasional mention of individuals whose stutter was totally absent when they spoke near the base of a waterfall.

Many explanations have been developed to account for this "waterfall phenomenon." Some feel that the loud noise serves as a distraction, while others say that it somehow leads the stutterer to conclude that his words will not be heard, and this in turn reduces stress and produces fluency.

This phenomenon formed the theoretical basis for the development by a team of researchers at the University of Edinburgh of an electronic device known, appropriately, as the "Edinburgh Masker." The principle of its operation is quite simple. A microphone is attached to the patient's neck by an elastic band. When the vocal cords start to vibrate, the vibration is detected by the microphone and the impulses are sent to a small device known as a white noise generator. White noise sounds very much like hissing steam. As soon as the white noise generator receives the impulses from the throat microphone, it becomes activated and the sound is amplified and sent through earphones worn by the patient.

This creates the following situation: When the patient is silent, the noise is off and he can hear the speech of others around him. As soon as he starts to speak, the noise comes on and it is loud enough that *he is unable to hear himself.* This tends to stop stuttering, but the price the patient must pay is obvious. First, there is the paraphernalia that must be worn at all times: a throat microphone, an amplifier, a noise generator, earphones, and the associated wiring to connect them. The patient is also obviously dependent on batteries and the hope that they do not run out in the middle of a conversation. Second, there is some evidence to suggest a possibility of nerve damage to the hearing nerves when there is prolonged exposure to loud noise. And third, there is the difficulty associated with phone conversations, since the earphones do not permit the convenient placement of the telephone against the ear.

There is one other serious problem associated with the device. The noise generator comes on initially after the first sound is produced, but as we have discovered, the locking of the vocal cords occurs before speech begins. And so the Masker is inoperative during the critical pre-speech period. The result is that the cords are still free to lock. In order to deal with that problem, one is often forced to use a starter such as a brief humming sound to get the Masker going.

The principle behind the Masker is an admirable one. The waterfall effect is real. The reason it works, however, did not come to light until recently. The hearing nerve, as it courses to the brain, attaches to the nerves coming up from the vocal cords. There is a commingling of fibers and impulses. When a loud noise is presented to the ears, a very strong signal comes up the hearing nerve, and when this signal commingles with the vocal cords' nerve signals it alters them. This altered signal is no longer the correct stimulus for triggering stuttering—and no stutter occurs.

In the future, small implantable devices will be placed in

the middle ear to accomplish the same end. They will make use of the hearing nerve to intercept the impulses coming up from the vocal-cord nerves so that the impulses no longer have cue value to elicit stuttering.

IT IS clear that what every stutterer in the world is looking for is an expeditious cure—a cure that requires no effort. The prospects for the future are thus particularly appealing because they are passive. Apart from presenting himself for treatment, the patient is not called upon to participate in any way in his recovery. In addition, the treatment usually requires a single intervention and the recovery period is short.

It is my belief that by the year 2000 some of these approaches will begin to be manifest. Research is well under way and knowledge is accumulating at a rapid rate. The next chapter in the treatment of stuttering will probably read, "Stuttering: Its Speedy, Total, and Permanent Cure."

Part III

SUCCESS STORIES

Now that you have learned about the treatment process, let's hear firsthand from just a few of the thousands of people who have succeeded in overcoming stuttering. What makes these first-person accounts extraordinary is not only their inherent drama, but the fact that they were told before a large audience as after-dinner speeches.

18 *The Computer Professional*

I REMEMBER a childhood friend asking me why I talked funny sometimes. The question surprised me, but it was the beginning of an awareness that I did have difficulty speaking at times. This was at the age of eight. I soon realized that I was having difficulty in school particularly, and was enrolled in speech therapy for the first time in the second grade. I met other children with the same problem at the institute. I attended therapy sessions for over a year, but I'm not sure what effect it had.

By the third grade I had begun to experience real humiliation and frustration in classroom reading situations. Reading and speaking before a group became an experience to be feared. I was aware of laughter as I stuttered my way through repetitious sentences. Words on a page would blur before my eyes and lose their meaning. The harder I tried, the more my fluency disintegrated. The next few years were the worst. I considered pretending to be a mute as a way of avoiding the uncontrollable stuttering which was causing me embarrassment and shame. I had heard someone say that I would outgrow it eventually, and this was the hope I held on to.

I remember a period of several months when speech

without stuttering was impossible. I clung to a few short answers which I felt safe in saying: "Same here" and "I don't know" were a couple.

I began to substitute words and phrases for those I knew would cause me trouble, and gradually built up a fairly successful ability for scanning and switching to improve fluency. Of course, there were still unavoidable situations in which I could not substitute, and the blockages were interminable at times. An article I had to read to the class as a freshman in high school is still fresh in my mind. It dealt with abbreviations and acronyms used for agencies and companies. It took me great lengths of time to stutter through the letters which appeared over and over again. I managed to get through part of the first page before the laughter was apparent. I would have laughed myself if I hadn't felt so miserable. I finally looked at the teacher in such a pleading way that he had someone else finish reading for me.

At home, things were little better. I dreaded the use of the phone. It was something I used only under duress. To be home alone and hear the phone ring was traumatic. Each time I faced a decision to just let it ring or force myself to pick up the receiver. Inevitably, when I did answer it, my stuttering was disastrous.

As a teenager, I still felt I would outgrow my affliction. I couldn't imagine being a stuttering adult. As a sophomore in high school I decided to return to the institute for therapy. After several months of group therapy I still didn't understand what we were doing, what we were trying to do, or whether I was improving. I stopped going.

I chose a technical area of study in college, since it was clear to myself and my counselors that I would function best where oral communication would not be a burden. I periodically reviewed the literature on speech therapy for hints and theories relating to my problem. I realized that I was not going to outgrow it after all, and tried to plan accordingly.

As an adult, my pattern was still to avoid people and situations which gave me trouble. I was quite fluent at times. The phone remained an obstacle. Extreme nausea, rapid heartbeat, sweating, and shortness of breath were some of my reactions to simple phone calls. Clever substitutions and various distractions (for example, writing words on a chalkboard) got me through many situations. Some friends of mine were unaware that I had a problem. They could never guess the energy and planning I put in to keep my speech "under control."

About a year ago, my parents sent me a book on the airflow technique. I was curious enough to read it. I became excited as I saw my frustrations catalogued and explained in those pages. Understanding the problem was almost satisfaction enough; I was hesitant at first to commit myself to the possibility of undergoing therapy. I finally resolved that if I were ever to try to beat stuttering again, this was the opportunity. I arranged for treatment knowing that if it failed, it would not be from lack of effort on my part.

At the end of the first day of treatment and practice I felt that the technique did in fact give me control over my speech for the first time. The first night during treatment was very restless, my subconscious perhaps refusing to admit what I already sensed. From the first day, I ceased to struggle against vocal-cord locks. I learned to recognize them and to respond with careful use of technique. I dedicated myself to using the technique correctly and at all times. The prescribed practice became my top priority when I returned home and began the follow-up phase of therapy. With the help of my family at home and an understanding supervisor at work, I was able to follow the program faithfully.

I still encountered occasional blocks in high-stress situations, invariably due to sloppy use of the technique. As my command of the technique grew, my confidence increased, and in situation by situation I was successful.

Word substitution was the first crutch I discarded. It took me a while to get used to always saying exactly what I originally intended to say.

By the fourth month of therapy, the phone was no longer an object of fear. I was now pleased to hear it ring, since it would present an opportunity to further practice my technique. The apprehension and former stress symptoms were gone.

By the sixth month, I knew that I could be completely successful if I kept at it. I had already been through some serious high-stress experiences with total fluency. I was having no problems with group situations, interviews, or phone calls.

The most difficult part has been to develop a high degree of concentration on the technique, regardless of my surroundings. Diligent practice and effort make it possible. There were some early instances in which another speaker or questioner would become impatient for a reply. I learned to not react to this, but to still take a second or so to employ the technique. It amazed me that no one ever realized that a flow was being employed unless I specifically demonstrated it for them. Some people did indicate they thought I was speaking a little slower than usual.

I think I can best categorize the therapy as a learning process. I didn't become totally fluent overnight, but each day has increased the range of situations in which fluency is achieved, regardless of stress level.

At the age of thirty-five, I have started a new phase in my life. There are many things I have done during the last year which were quite beyond me before, simple things like ordering over the phone, calling the hospital in an emergency, inquiring about a new position, speaking easily to people—always a problem in the past.

I achieved a goal of teaching in my church, something I had long hoped to be able to do.

I changed jobs during the therapy, taking a position

requiring constant interaction with people under situations of considerable stress.

I have been able to eliminate the dependency I had on others to help me through situations, either voluntarily or by manipulation on my part. I feel that others can now count on me, and I can offer the kind of support and leadership I once shied away from.

19 *The Importer*

I was a dropout before I started. The National Center for Stuttering wouldn't take me on as a patient because they felt my stress level was too high to do the airflow technique effectively. But having seen the technique work (on me) during my interview, I knew I had to take the workshop. So NCS agreed to have a therapist monitor me for a few weeks to see if I could handle it. I started the training a month later.

My life up till then was a constant inner battle of trying to hide the fact I was a stutterer from everyone—somewhere along the way I got the impression people looked upon us as mentally deficient. So at all costs I had to hide my speech problem and became a "closet stutterer." How successful I was didn't really matter; it was hardly worth the effort. In fact had I come out in the open and admitted to myself and others I was in fact a stutterer, life would have been a whole lot easier for me, and later on it would have been easier to control. I didn't get involved in lengthy conversations; I avoided every talking situation possible; I didn't order what I wanted in restaurants; people always phoned for me; school was a worse horror for me because I wasn't very apt at substituting one word for another at that time. And worst of all, when I did stutter, which was more often than I like to admit, it left terrible pains in my body and mind, and left me feeling helpless.

Of course, I went to all the speech helpers and quacks available at the time, from therapists to hypnotists. Nothing helped. To avoid talking in certain situations, I would go as far as forcing a self-inflicted sore throat so I could legitimately cancel any speaking assignments. I could write and make a speech without stuttering if the vowel sound was hooked on to a consonant making it one word—like: "Can I havea canof beer?" I can recall hundreds of stories in my youth and mature years where, as a result of my stuttering, I did not lead a normal life—and I was very bitter about it. It never fully left me.

I was all through with speech doctors and their cures so even the NCS method held no interest for me—until one night while coming up from the basement I called my wife's name, but never got it out. Instead I fell over backwards on the stairs, going into a beautiful spasm and nearly breaking my neck. I just grabbed the bannister in time. That convinced me to give it one more shot. Her name? Ellen!

I can never forget when my therapist took me into a cafeteria and encouraged me to use the airflow technique speaking to total strangers. For the first time in my life I spoke without faking it and without stuttering. I put my arms around him and couldn't speak because of the excitement of *being able to speak*.

20 *The Seminary Student*

As FAR back as I can remember, I've always stuttered. I remember early in childhood, asking members of my family why. I was never satisfied with their answers. One interesting theory was that it was due to my frustration over a toy fire engine. I was two years old, and the fire engine was too big for me. My feet could not touch the pedals, and it was suggested that I became extremely frustrated in my attempts to make the fire engine move forward. As a result of this frustration, I began to stutter. Whatever merit this theory may have, I've learned not to speculate. Suffice to say that much of my early childhood was spent trying to solve the riddle of my stuttering problem.

Because I stuttered, I had a very frustrating childhood. On a scale from one to ten (ten being the worst), I would rate my childhood stuttering at about a six, with gusts to eight. I believe I was a normal kid, with average abilities in most areas. But because of my stuttering, I was alienated from potential friends and opportunities. I developed a tendency to frown which has plagued me most of my life. Even today, I am generally regarded as being unfriendly because of my tendency to look cross.

I have suffered educationally because of my stuttering. I would have done anything to keep from contributing orally during class, or from formally giving oral reports.

I would even refrain from asking questions, or sometimes I would pretend not to know the answers to questions if I was called on. All of this dodging during school tended to keep my grades down in the average category. I believe now I could have earned much higher marks had I not stuttered.

As I embarked on high school days, I entered one of the most frustrating times in my life. Much of the normal high school life is social in nature, and I felt alienated from most of it. I never did much dating during those years because I was too afraid to talk to any girls. I was sort of blacklisted from the "in crowd" because of my stuttering.

One particular incident captures the frustration and embarrassment of my high school days. It occurred in my English class during my junior year. There were a couple of guys in the class I had been hanging around with, and I really wanted to be friends with them. I had been making strenuous efforts to keep my stuttering to a minimum around them. As part of a class assignment, we were to team up into small groups, and give oral reports on a short novel. I was teamed up with my two "friends." As you might imagine, this proved to be one of the most embarrassing situations I have ever faced.

We got up before the class, and we each gave our portion of the report. I was the last to give his report, and I was tied up in knots in anticipation. I started my report in a very choppy manner, and then I lost all composure. I suddenly locked on a feared word, and I couldn't break the lock. I just stood there in front of the class, and I groaned on like an automobile trying to start on a cold morning. My face turned many shades of red, and I believe I did some slobbering as well. Before I was done, I had locked on several other words, and as I walked back to my seat, I remember myself as a very humiliated young man. I also never seemed to click with those two "friends" after that.

I have been frustrated with several "therapies." I remember in grade school, once a week I went to a school therapist. This was a frustrating experience because I never did much stuttering in front of the therapist. I remember when I was in junior high, my mother took me to the family doctor. I did not stutter at all in front of him either, but he prescribed "tranquilizers" as part of my therapy. He said that this was "the newest thing." I never felt the "tranquilizers" helped at all. More recently, I went to the speech therapist at the university I am now attending. Among other things, she said I should do relaxing exercises, and I should slow my speech down in stress situations. I feel this particular therapist helped somewhat, but I still felt frustrated and helpless. She could not adequately explain to me why I stuttered, and the best she could offer me was minor improvement over the rest of my life. She spoke in terms of "control" but not "cure." It seemed to be another Band-Aid approach to speech therapy.

I would like to relate at this time the events that led to finding out about the National Center for Stuttering's therapy program. By my early teens, I had learned to be apathetic about my speech problem. I decided the less I said, the better off I would be. In fact, in my late teens I even used alcohol and drugs excessively, partly because they relaxed me and I didn't stutter as much. However, I was jolted from my apathy at the age of twenty, when I received Christ into my life. I could no longer tolerate staying quiet. I had to tell others about what He had done for me.

I found out it is pretty tough to be a witness for my faith with a speech impediment, however. I also began to realize I wanted to begin to train to become a Christian minister. I knew that something had to be done to improve my speech.

My parents saw an article in a Long Beach newspaper which told of the amazing work that the National Center for Stuttering was doing in the area of stuttering therapy.

They ordered a book which described the program. After reading it I knew this was the answer to the problem. Here was a therapy which pinpointed the physical mechanism of stuttering, and which set about to attack the problem source. This was definitely not a Band-Aid approach to speech therapy. After reading the book, I contacted the center and signed up for one of their seminars on the West Coast.

The seminar in San Francisco was two full days of intense therapy. I left San Francisco on cloud nine, knowing the airflow technique was going to work. And it has! But I do not wish to paint a completely rosy picture. Old habits die hard, and stuttering is definitely a set of bad speaking habits. The power of stuttering seems to be in the fear of speaking. Fear is a powerful thing. That is why, as a necessary part of therapy, we have a set of practice exercises to perform each day, to make the new airflow technique more natural than the old habit of locking the vocal cords and stuttering. It takes discipline to do the exercise that is needed everyday. But the rewards are definitely worth it. I would estimate that I have attained about 95 percent fluency. Generally, if I encounter a problem, it is because I have not used the airflow technique properly. I must evaluate the failure, and then set about to correct the problem. I believe one of the strengths in the technique is that the ignorance about stuttering is replaced with knowledge. If problems are encountered, they are then to be analyzed and corrected.

I am convinced that 100 percent fluency is within my grasp. The airflow therapy has changed my life, given me the opportunity to help myself which is very exciting. I am looking to the future with confidence, not with fear, and I am forever indebted to the National Center for Stuttering.

21 *The Retired Mechanical Engineer*

MY CASE as a stutterer is unique in that I did nothing to correct it until I was seventy-four years of age. I stuttered mildly as a boy, but managed to get by without too much trouble. But after college, when I entered the business world, the situation worsened and I had my troubles. I attempted to speak freely using human willpower, but the result were disastrous. I developed ways of getting by. I often coughed to get started; I avoided certain words, especially those starting with the letter *s*, and this resulted in very odd sentence structure. Sometimes my telephone conversations were most embarrassing. I did a very bad job of introducing others, asking for directions, and ordering in restaurants. At times I wanted to run and hide.

But I didn't. I struggled on, learning to live with a condition which was so abnormal. I often thought of seeking some sort of therapy but never did. Now I am just as satisfied that I didn't, because having talked recently with other stutterers who tried various curative systems, I learned that none of them were helpful.

I had a fairly successful business career in spite of my handicap, although I surely could have done better had my speech been normal.

Then, about twelve months ago I read an article on stuttering, which described briefly the airflow technique. This intrigued me, and I arranged to join an NCS workshop in Los Angeles.

After a revealing two days at the workshop, there began the (sometimes arduous) work of mastering the technique under any circumstance that can befall a speaker. Frankly, I had no idea a wrong habit of speaking could be so stubborn. It seems so easy to master the technique under controlled conditions, but oh, how easy it is to forget and return to the old habit. With the help of the weekly tapes reviewed by the National Center for Stuttering staff worker (bless her!), I am making slow but steady progress, and daily getting closer to the goal of complete correction of the old difficulty.

Proofs of progress are many. The automatic use of the technique is becoming stronger and stronger. Words starting with *s* give me practically no trouble. I use the telephone freely. I make introductions with ease. I order in restaurants for myself and others. I ask directions without difficulty. Speaking in public is becoming easier. I have given talks before more than a hundred people, and while not yet perfect, I have exhibited a freedom I never had before. I have not the slightest doubt my continued practice will bring about the elimination of the problem that plagued me so long.

To say that I am grateful is a complete understatement. When I recall the handicap I once had and note the freedom I now have, it seems like a miracle. And it is all so simple. It promises a wonderful boon to countless individuals who are now in bondage to this awful affliction.

22 *The Social Worker*

I REMEMBER vividly when I was seven years old (that was twenty-six years ago). My parents were vociferously affirming, "You are not really a stutterer, you just have to learn to think before you talk." This notion—that something was screwed up in my thought processes—set me on an incredible journey from therapist to therapist in search of a way, method, or system to tighten up my "sick" mind and help me to stop stuttering.

This poor, distorted self-image was continually reinforced by teachers and schoolmates. I remember the frequent instances of laughter in the elementary grades when I was called on to speak. I remember the feeling of utter terror going up and down my spine in anticipation of being singled out to speak. I remember the grimaces of disappointment on my father's face when I blocked on a word or phrase. His body language affected me greatly and usually released a bevy of verbal blocks. So at an early age I learned that if I wanted to passively upset my parents, all I had to do was stutter—and since I was very angry, I did it all the time.

Then the myriad of therapies began. First, it was from a matronly woman who lived in a house full of antiques. A classical speech therapist, she had me recite, curl my tongue, and massage my neck muscles. I lost interest in this quickly and besides receiving some candy canes I don't recall much benefit from the experience.

My next adventure was with an institute specializing in speech disorders. The modalities this time were group therapy, play therapy, and relaxation exercises. Imagine for a moment the painfully tedious progress which can be made in a group full of stutterers trying to communicate with each other. Time passed slowly but my symptoms held fast.

After a therapeutic hiatus of three or four years, I found myself an awkward adolescent with a horrible self-concept. I frankly thought I was crazy and persuaded my parents to have me see a psychiatrist. He was a classical analyst who delighted in relating my adolescent psycho-sexual fantasies to my stuttering. He tried to hypnotize me but I did not trust him and hence was a poor subject.

My social life was a disaster. Since I could not speak over the telephone, I found it very difficult to go out on dates. My friends occasionally made calls, pretending they were me, but as you can imagine, it was impossible to follow up on such proxy dates!

In high school I excelled in writing. I became editor of the literary magazine and was a speech writer for winning candidates in student government. I spoke vicariously through them.

In college the same social pressures and frustrations increased. I consequently did very poorly during the first two years and decided to have another round at psychotherapy. This time it was with a very supportive "ego psychologist." My fluency did not increase but I began to understand myself better and my self-esteem improved considerably. I decided to take a master's degree in social work and in graduate school I was an honor student.

Everything was going fine until a research project I was conducting required the use of a telephone for interviews. I manipulated the situation by getting my wife to call for me and even faking some interviews. The reality of living a lie threw me into a serious depression.

The "better living through chemistry" concept took firm hold of me via a team of organic psychiatrists attached to the university I was attending. In addition to antidepressants, they were experimenting with major tranquilizers to relax my neck muscles. I gave up that folly when I experienced the horror of not being able to swallow.

I dropped out of graduate school and went to a rural part of the western United States to work. I got a job as a school social worker. Since this job required considerable verbal ability, my newfound depression was a convenient out to continuing the job.

I went back into therapy—this time with a Jungian analyst. After five sessions he wisely told me to "stop achieving, drop out, and try to find yourself." At the same time I met a man who was deeply involved in the Synanon-type therapeutic community movement back East. I knew that if I were to really grow up I would have to rid myself of those drugs which the good doctors had prescribed for me. My wife and I flew back East and spent a miraculous two weeks of detoxification and self-discovery. My depression game was completely shattered by this community of ex-cons and recovered addicts.

We returned to the West and began an incredible drug-free adventure into the potentialities of the fulfillment of human consciousness and practical mysticism. Our lives were finally together and although I did stutter occasionally on the telephone and in groups, it did not seem to hamper my development. My spiritual master, Meher Baba, once said, "Do your best, then don't worry; be happy and leave the results to God." I took these words as my guide and was resigned to the fact that I would probably stutter the rest of my life. There's a funny thing about resignation. Once you are really resigned to something, it occasionally happens that opportunities for self-growth arise of which you had not previously been aware.

I noticed an article in a magazine about the airflow technique. Since my profession is the evaluation of clinical therapies I was quite skeptical of the reported high success rate, but I was intrigued enough to read the literature. My scientific side was quite satisfied and my metaphysical nature was equally pleased (mystics of all traditions have been aware of the power of the breath as a healing tool throughout the ages).

I entered therapy and on the following day spoke fluently! Now a year has gone by and I have been practicing daily on an intensive basis. I can honestly say that I remember only about ten occasions on which I have stuttered during the past year, and it was only when I forgot to conscientiously apply the technique.

I thank God for the wisdom of this technique and for my continued strength to harness the healing power of the breath.

Part IV

FINAL WORDS

23 *To the Stutterer*

IF YOU stutter and you've read this book this far, you've undoubtedly seen yourself described several times. You understand your form of stuttering and know how it developed. Perhaps you have experienced a rekindling of interest in doing something about your problem. You've likely had the traditional speech therapies and/or psychotherapies and know these are not the solution. The key, of course, is understanding, and what I have attempted to do in this book is relieve some of the mystery and ignorance surrounding stuttering. You may already have experienced a reduction in your overall stress as a result.

The treatment I have described may enable you to profit still further. Your stress may be so low you may be able to treat yourself. But *this book is not intended as a self-help manual*. Self-treatment is not advised. Many of the subtleties of the technique must be seen, and most patients tend to jump ahead too quickly in their practice regimen and invariably experience difficulty. If you are serious about addressing your problem, call the National Stutterers' Hotline at 1-800-221-2483 for further information about your therapy options.

Motivation will be your most important asset. If you feel compelled to seek therapy only because of outside pressures from family and friends, you will be approaching this experience from the wrong direction. The decision must be a personal one, for the work, while not difficult, requires faith and determination. You will have to make a major commitment to restructuring a part of your speech. Learning the airflow technique is not difficult; using it in all speaking situations and extinguishing the fears that lie in the way is the real challenge.

Most of us take speech for granted. You are used to the struggling and the avoidance behaviors associated with your stuttering, even though they are physically and psychologically exhausting. But if you have a specific goal in mind—whether finding a new career, or seeking advancement in your present one, or simply freeing yourself of this nagging constraint so that you can become a new person—you will find the strength to break out of your old habit and sustain your motivation as you acquire and build your new one.

Thousands of stutterers have received airflow training. The long-term success rate in our most recent published report is 93.4 percent (see the Appendix). This high rate of success may appear startling in view of the poor results reported in the research literature of the past. But if you simply reread this book, you will understand why airflow therapy has achieved such excellent results. The therapy is based on a theory which does a better job of accounting for stuttering than any previous theory. The therapy is a direct, logical outcome of the theory and involves not only a set of techniques, but also the patient's understanding of how his stuttering began and why the technique is effective. This understanding is crucial to the outcome and accounts in large measure for the virtually negligible incidence of relapse.

When I explain the cause of stuttering to patients the usual response is, "You know, that makes sense. It agrees with what I had always felt. I knew I wasn't crazy or neurotic." It is my sincerest hope that this is how you feel having read this book. The evidence, based upon the results of work with thousands of people like yourself, is on your side.

24 *To Friends and Family*

Just about everyone knows someone who stutters. Perhaps it's the young man at the gas station, or the boy who delivers the newspapers, or the English teacher you had in high school. Or perhaps it's your brother, your uncle, or your best friend. How do you feel when you see and hear them stutter? Probably you want to help. And perhaps you do by providing the word they are so desperately struggling to say.

You've always wished someone would tell you how to react when you're around someone who stutters. But no one does. Like many, you think it is a "psychological" problem, or that "their thoughts are running faster than their words." Whatever it is, you know one thing for sure: their stuttering makes you uncomfortable.

You've tried to ignore it. You've maintained eye contact and kept an even expression on your face. Pretending it isn't there seems to be the only course of action. After all, what can you say or do to help?

Imagine the following scene. A stutterer is talking to you. He is under stress, tensing, and blocking severely while he is pretending nothing's wrong. You, the listener are also stressed, tense, and also pretending nothing's wrong. Neither you nor he says anything; both of you suffer as you remain locked in a socially-prescribed vise of denial.

Now imagine a different scene, in a make-believe world. In this world there is a law which dictates that if you see someone stuttering, you are required to immediately go up to that person and say, "Just a minute now, breathe in, let some air out passively, and slow the first word." In this make-believe world everyone knows about the locking of the vocal cords, everyone knows about a suitable means for preventing the locking, and everyone knows that instead of saying nothing when you see someone stutter, you should immediately go up to the person and give what is generally recognized to be the right correcting information. Furthermore, everyone who stutters knows, from the time they are children, that every time they stutter everyone within earshot will come up to them and give the right correcting information. How much stuttering would there be? Not very much!

If the President of the United States addressed the public on television, he could give the right correcting information for stuttering in thirty seconds, and suddenly 2.6 million Americans would find their lives much improved.

Well, that is not about to happen, but you can do the next best thing. You can let people who stutter know that there has been a revolution in the understanding and treatment of stuttering. Most stutterers simply aren't aware of the advances in the field of stuttering. They've given up; they've had therapies years ago which didn't work, and now they've joined the conspiracy of denial. They deserve to be able to consider the possibility of living a normal existence. And you can help.

You can start by reading this book and becoming informed about the nature of the problem and the options available in therapy. Then share the news with someone who stutters. If it is awkward for you to go up to a stutterer and just start talking about his problem, then contact the National Center for Stuttering and we will send him this book or a packet of free information. There is no place for timidity and reticence when you think of the desperate conditions under which the average stutterer functions.

Remember that the stutterer has spent years learning to stutter, and that unlearning this habit, including all the fears associated with it, will take time too. Your encouragement and support as an enlightened friend or family member will be essential to the stutterer's success in overcoming his affliction.

On numerous occasions patients have come to my office for evaluation carrying a yellowed newspaper clipping about the center—sent to them years earlier by an interested friend or relative, and acted upon only now, in a moment of personal crisis. The fact that they kept the article and didn't throw it away, carried it continuously in a wallet or purse, suggests that the underlying desire to solve the problem has always been there.

When I asked one patient why she had waited so long to receive treatment, she said, "Doctor, I've had so many disappointments in the past, I was afraid to hope." Help rekindle that hope by sharing this book with someone who stutters.

25 *To the Therapist*

H<small>ERE</small> I want to offer some cautionary advice to speech therapists.

The airflow technique differs in important ways from speech therapy. As is apparent from the success of this technique, focusing on the speech problem itself has been one of the major mistakes in the treatment of stuttering. The struggle which so characterizes the disorder is not with speech, but rather against a locking of the vocal cords which has occurred just prior to speech. Therefore attempting to work on speech is a grave mistake, and any form of therapy that uses this approach is of dubious value.

Traditional speech therapy techniques such as "bounce," "pull-out," and "cancellation" have no value in the treatment program presented in this book. Our attention, and the attention of our patients, must be constantly focused upon what they do *before* they speak. If they set themselves up properly, that is, use the passive airflow and slow their first word, their speech will emerge fluently. This preoccupation with preparation and a total disregard for speech constitutes the major distinction between airflow therapy and traditional speech therapy.

It should come as no surprise, then, to discover that I often begin lectures to speech therapists with this statement: "Speech therapy does not work in the treatment of stuttering, but speech therapists, when properly trained, are probably the best people to work with stutterers."

The National Center for Stuttering has developed a training program for speech clinicians which is now available in many cities across the United States. The training program consists of both observation and practice. In the first phase, therapists observe a two-day intensive treatment workshop. The second phase follows the workshop and consists of a six-month clinical application of the therapeutic techniques demonstrated during the workshop. Therapists administer airflow therapy to their own patients, recording on tape their initial presentation and periodic therapy sessions. These tapes are then mailed to the center for evaluation. All tapes are returned with comments and suggestions.

At the end of the six-month monitoring phase, those therapists demonstrating a thorough understanding of the airflow technique and the ability to transfer that understanding in the therapeutic setting are awarded certification.

The center has maintained a training program for speech clinicians for more than fourteen years. Typically, the center trains about two hundred clinicians a year. Since there are more than sixty thousand speech therapists in the United States, however, much work clearly remains to be done.

APPENDIX

A Study of the Long-term Effects of a Multidimensional Treatment Program for Stutterers

THE PURPOSE of this study is to present data relevant to the long-term effects of the multidimensional treatment program described in this book. The results are based upon a population of 625 patients who participated in the NCS program.

Subjects

The experimental population was composed of 492 males (mean age, 31.6 years) and 133 females (mean age, 27.4). Almost all had had speech therapy or psychotherapy at some point in their lives prior to enrolling in the NCS program. For 538 patients, their overt struggle symptoms ranged from mild to severe; for 87 patients, there were no overt struggle behaviors, but rather a well-developed word-substitution capability. This group, labeled "closet stutterers," was comprised of 62 females and 25 males.

Method
Each patient was treated using the methods described in this book. All received weekly individualized assignments and sent tape cassettes to their therapist at the center on an average of at least once every ten days during the follow-up period. All were required to attend local club meetings or to communicate regularly by telephone with fellow patients in their area. All attended at least two regularly scheduled refresher courses.

Prior to and at the end of the follow-up period (one year) the patients were called upon to complete a detailed questionnaire. The questionnaire was a self-assessment of relative percent speaking success in each of twelve representative speaking situations. The test was also readministered after twenty-four and thirty-six months to determine the effects of posttreatment years upon the groups' judgments of their performance.

Results
At the end of the initial twelve-month period, 96 percent of the patients reported that the program had been successful. One year after termination of therapy, at twenty-four months, the success rate had dropped to 93 percent.

Discussion
The definition of success used in this study was "to be essentially symptom-free in all daily routine speaking situations." There was no attempt to define success as total elimination of undesirable habits; rather it was defined in a functional sense—that is, to function routinely without stuttering, word- or sound-substituting, or avoiding speaking situations.

Might the patients slip once in a while and stutter? The answer is yes. But they could recover immediately and, most importantly, reported that they were not psychologically devastated by the block. They knew it was caused by a failure to employ technique and further knew they could take immediate action to prevent further blocks from occurring.

Thus, the results of this study indicate that for adults, well over nine out of ten can expect to have a relatively permanent success with the techniques described— provided that they are religious in their adherence to all aspects of the program.

But what of the "failures"? It depends how failure is defined. For example, one of the patients, a stockbroker, entered the program, performed well during the initial phase, followed that by entering a telephone hierarchy, spent an unusually long time going through the hierarchy (four months), practiced several other hierarchies to success, and at nine months, quit. When tested, both at twelve and twenty-four months, the patient was still stuttering in some situations but reported overall that he personally considered the program a success. He revealed that his major, if not sole, purpose in entering the program had been to become fluent on the telephone since, if fluent, he could call new customers and be expected to increase his income substantially. The excessive amount of time spent on the telephone hierarchy was therefore a reflection of his personal emphasis. His business had increased significantly and, although he was stuttering in a number of situations, he had achieved his major goal. The program had performed its function for him. It was a success.

Many patients, after improving substantially in a number of speaking situations, are quite content with their accomplishment and simply stop practicing. There may be several situations in which they have consistent difficulty, but these occur for them so infrequently or are so relatively unimportant that the motivation for continued practice is nonexistent. These individuals are pleased with their result, though from our research point of view are considered part of the "nonsuccess" group.

The slippage of three percentage points between the twelve- and twenty-four-month assessments represented approximately 20 individuals who reported the reoccurrence of difficulty in some speaking situations. All 625 patients had been without formal therapy for a year, and it was surprising to find such a small number reporting difficulty. It was possible to reinitiate treatment for 11 of the patients, and after a month all had recovered to their twelve-month levels. These results suggest that a small group of patients may require some form of periodic refresher course for a period beyond the formal year of practice.

One important additional result emerged from the study: the likelihood of relapse appears to be great in the first five months of treatment. During this time the patients are fragile, and a high-stress episode can provoke an onset of stuttering that, if left unchecked, can result in a disastrous downward performance spiral. We have discovered that the support groups, hot lines, weekly monitorings, and refresher courses have saved dozens of patients from relapse. The conclusion is inescapable that all treatment programs must provide these services if patients are to achieve comparable levels of success.

Acknowledgments

I WISH to acknowledge those responsible for the production of this book: George Gray, my high school teacher, whose inspiring lectures persuaded me to march to the rhythm of a different drummer; Colin Wilson, author of *The Outsider*, who, along with Robert Frost and Ayn Rand convinced me that I was right in choosing "the road less traveled"; John Black, professor of speech science at Ohio State University, who exposed me to the beauty of nature through science, a discipline that enabled me to discover the physical cause of stuttering; Lorraine Schneider, my colleague at the National Center for Stuttering, who as my perfect foil consistently tempered an often precipitous enthusiasm with the cool detachment of reason; my editor, Fred Hills, and his assistant, Daphne Bien, who transformed my manuscript into a readable book; my wife, Judith, who endured the deprivations that come with a life of travel and service. And to my patients who, with unending patience, educated me about stuttering.

Index

142   *Index*

larynx, 14, 52
learned behavior, 16, 18, 19;
    stuttering as, 17–19, 22, 50,
    129
Levinson, Steve, 64

men vs. women, stuttering in,
    22, 35
meridians, acupressure, 73
monitor system, 86, 136, 138
MotivAider, 64–65
motor nerves, vocal cord, 98–
    100
mouth breathing, 58
muscle relaxant drugs, 50
muscle tension, 21; relaxation
    therapies, 45, 50, 80; in
    vocal cords, normal, 28,
    52; in vocal cords of stut-
    terers, 14, 21–22, 28–29,
    53, 96

name, stutter problems with,
    24–25, 71–72
National Center for Stuttering
    (NCS), 33, 58, 79, 81, 82,
    88, 93–94, 96, 110–11, 114–
    115, 117; certification of
    therapists by, 95, 131; re-
    search at, 98; training pro-
    gram for speech clinicians,
    131; treatment program
    results, 135–38
National Institute of Deafness
    and Communication Disor-
    ders, 97
National Institutes of Health,
    97
National Stutterers' Hotline,
    83–84, 93, 125
nerves, vocal cord, 18, 98; in-
    jections into, 98–100
New York University, 99; Medi-
    cal Center, 13
nonverbal behavior of stutter-
    ers, 16–17, 18–19, 32–33;
    closet stutterers, 35–37, 39

outgrowing stuttering, 88–89;
    probability factor, 89–90, 93

passive airflow, 51–56; *see also*
    airflow technique
phobias, Callahan treatment of,
    73–76
physical basis of stuttering, 13–
    14, 15, 21–22, 51
play therapy, 119
primary stuttering, 39–41; treat-
    ment of, 41–42
probability outgrowth factor,
    89–90, 93
progressive relaxation, 45
prolongations, 15, 17, 30
psychological triggers of stut-
    tering, 23–29, 51; tradi-
    tional view, 19, 20–21
psychotherapy, 20–21, 125, 135
public speaking, 24; in work-
    shops, 58; *see also* speaking
    situations
punishment therapy, 48–49

real-world exercises, 66–67
refined sugar, in diet, 91
refresher courses, 82–83, 136,
    138
relapse, 77–78, 81, 82, 95; pre-
    venting, 79–80; rarity of,
    126; time of greatest risk
    of, 138
relaxation therapies, 45–46, 50,
    114, 119; bathtub tech-
    nique, 79–80
repetitions, 15, 17, 30, 39, 40
research, 97–102
respiration, *see* breathing
rubber-tube feedback device,
    58, 59

scanning habit, 40–41, 67, 68,
    82; case history, 106
school, problems in, 92
secondary stuttering, 39–41;
    treatment of, 42